NURSING, YES I DO

NURSING, YES I DO!

In Honor of Nurses Everywhere

Aubrey Labalia

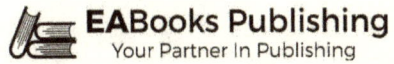

Nursing, Yes I Do! In honor of nurses everywhere.
Copyright @ 2024 Aubrey Labalia

All rights reserved. No part of this publication may be reproduced or transmitted in any form or by any electronic or mechanical means including photo copying, recording, or any information storage and retrieval system now known or to be invented, without permission in writing from the publisher or the author.

Cover design: Robin Black
Cover photo: iStockphoto/sellen
Back cover photo: iStock-sudok1

ISBN: 978-1-955309-93-6
LCCN: 2024900127

Published by EA Books Publishing, a division of
Living Parables of Central Florida, Inc. a 501c3

EABooksPublishing.com

ACKNOWLEDGMENTS

This book would not have come to fruition if not for the kind and talented people I worked with and collaborated with.

Without my husband and children offering their support to move forward with this book, I may have never finished it.

I am forever grateful to the dedicated nurses I had the pleasure of working with. Some of those very same nurses taught me not only the medical aspects of nursing but also the means to deal with patients, families, and colleagues.

From there, I am appreciative of the help from two authors who provided me with the resources to author a book and fine-tune my writing skills.

One of the resources referred to me was Word Weavers. They are a group of seasoned authors welcoming those less seasoned and or newbies to educate and enhance their writing skills. I found their method of critiquing in a group setting extremely beneficial.

Lastly, a special thank you to EA Publishing for their guidance and assistance in publishing my book.

DISCLAIMER

The medical and insurance-related information presented is general in nature and should not be used as a substitute for the advice of a physician and medical insurance company.

PREFACE

Suffering, whether physical or mental, is a constant in our life on this earth, so it's appropriate for each of us to do what we can to minimize distress. Perhaps no one does this more than nurses. Putting on a uniform and being part of a team that helps a sick person achieve wellness brings a sense of accomplishment and joy to one's heart.

Wrapping my stethoscope around my neck felt like winning a gold medal. This piece of equipment can identify preliminary problems with a patient's heart, lungs, and bowels. On top of that, when you help someone get well, you develop a relationship with them that is unlike any other.

Nurses often carry their helping mentality outside of their workspaces. I cannot tell you how many times I have been told by strangers after a brief conversation, "You must be a nurse."

I proudly reply, "Yes, I am."

People who don't spend a lot of time in medical settings get most of their ideas about nursing and healthcare from television shows and movies. Those characters and stories have a real impact on our beliefs. But when was the last time you read a book, saw a movie, or watched a TV show about nurses? Many movies and TV shows depict one or more heroic doctors treating their patients, with nurses as mere sidekicks.

Nurse Jackie aired on Showtime from 2009 to 2015. While I respect the acting abilities of the lead actress, the character turned me off. While she was a well-respected nurse, she dealt with drug addiction. It certainly brought excitement to the story, but did not represent the kind of real, dedicated nurses I've worked with.

Most recently, the Canadian TV series *Nurses* aired on NBC beginning in January 2020. The story surrounds five young nurses with a variety of personalities working at a busy hospital in downtown Toronto. The storyline has potential, however although it is reportedly renewed for a third season in Canada, its availability in the United States is uncertain.

Although the Covid pandemic showed many people the importance of nursing in healthcare, nurses are often still seen as bedpan handlers. In actuality, a nurse conducts the tasks of a personal care aide, nutritionist, teacher, phlebotomist, physical or occupational therapist, respiratory therapist, and social worker. And more.

To help give people a better picture of what nursing really looks like, I'm sharing the first thirty years of my nursing experiences. Names, genders, dates, and locations have been altered for HIPAA compliance and other personal privacy concerns.

Although much of the technology and some of the treatments have changed since my nursing career began in 1977, I hope that my story will increase awareness of the seriousness of our nursing shortage, encourage young people to enter this challenging career for the right reasons, and inspire the respect our nurses deserve. Ultimately, though, what I most want to accomplish is a positive impact on patient care, since that is of utmost importance.

Chapter One

FIRST YEAR OF NURSING SCHOOL

Our trainer, a tightly wound prima donna, spoke in a dull monotone as she walked up and down the rows of students. Although I was a high school junior, that day I wasn't at school. I was in training to be a salesclerk at Collette's Department Store. The store had a bare, gray-walled classroom in the back.

At one point, without meaning to, I yawned.

The trainer stopped in front of me. "Am I boring you?"

I sat up straighter. "No, ma'am." But I couldn't help but think, *Yep, lady, you are.*

The department store job would do for a while, and I enjoyed working with several other students at Collette's. But I really wanted to become a nurse. I had been interested in nursing since the eighth grade—I had even written a paper and had given a presentation on the topic. I often thought about the many different roles that nurses fill. Maybe that's why I was eventually driven to various healthcare positions.

I worked at the store during the last two years of high school and the two years of my nursing program. I earned $2.95 an hour, when the minimum wage was $2. That income helped supplement my parents' contribution to my schooling and gave me spending money. The store gave employees a twenty percent discount, so I bought clothes for my family and myself. Eventually, though, the novelty wore off, and I found myself eager to begin my nursing career.

My routine was school all day Monday through Friday, then I worked about twenty-five hours a week and did schoolwork until the wee hours of the morning. In between, I tried to have a social life.

In June of 1975, I graduated from high school and, at the end of our ceremony, tossed my cap as high as I could. My ambition was to move out of my hometown of Bastille to spread my wings, but for family reasons I remained local. This included attending Christolette College, a Catholic college.

Only about sixty students were enrolled in the nursing school. Half of them were fresh out of high school, and the other half had worked somewhere in the medical field and were furthering their careers. Only about four students were men. I valued the elder students and found them to be a great resource with the extensive homework and studying in this nursing program. It took twice as much time as it had in high school work.

Christolette College had a dorm where about fifteen students lived. My family lived in the city, close enough to campus that I walked to school. But I still heard the dorm residents' stories of the pranks they played on the nuns.

The convent was connected to the dorm, separated only by a door, which was hardly ever locked. This allowed the nuns to visit the students at will and vice versa. One time the dorm students snuck into the convent, stole a nun's bra, and put it in the freezer. And if students did not want the nuns to check their room, a little petroleum jelly on the doorknob did the trick.

Classroom Clinical Time

One of the first things one learns in nursing school is how to make a bed. That might sound overly simple, except when you have to do it while a person is still in it.

CHAPTER ONE FIRST YEAR OF NURSING SCHOOL

Mrs. Offenheimer was our primary classroom instructor—a vision of a nurse post–World War II, with her tightly curled black hair, slender build, and bright red lipstick. She was strictly business-minded, but fair.

The initial tasks she gave us were to make an unoccupied and occupied bed. In the past, the beds had to be made so tight that a quarter would bounce off the surface. Several years after WWII, this practice ended. Thank heaven for that—we all passed making the unoccupied bed after our first attempt.

For the occupied bed changing, I was partners with Corrine. She was tall and slender, with tightly cut short brown hair and sea green eyes. Her demeanor was sweet, and she was more private about her personal life than the rest of us.

I flipped a coin to determine if I would be the patient or the nurse: heads for patient and tails for the nurse. It was tails.

Corrine got into the bed, all six feet of her, and I listened to Mrs. Offenheimer's instructions on how to turn the patient.

"Stand on the side of the bed you are changing. Turn the patient away from you by placing the arm closest to you over their chest and bend the knee closest to you over the other leg."

I moved Corrine's limbs as instructed, while she tried to stay limp. I had to stifle a giggle.

"Gently roll the patient away from you," Mrs. Offenheimer said, "and start changing the bed. Make sure they have a side rail to grab onto, so you do not lose the patient on the floor. Repeat this by standing on the other side to complete the bed."

I did as she said and received a positive nod from Mrs. Offenheimer. Corrine and I switched roles. It is a little weird the first time you have your body manipulated by someone else, but this is one of the first lessons because it's so vital to patient care to do it correctly. You would be amazed how easy it is to do this even with an extremely obese patient.

Corrine also received a positive nod. Our classmate Andrea, however, was not so lucky. She was partnered with Bob. Andrea and Bob were not much older than me, and this was their first healthcare experience.

Bob was a large man—not obese, but much larger than Andrea. As she rolled Bob toward the other side of the bed, he grasped the side rail.

The rail thunked downward—it wasn't locked in place. Bob rolled right off the bed and onto the floor. As he rolled, he took the sheets with him. That kind of cushioned the fall—somewhat.

We all gasped in shock.

Still tangled in sheets, Bob staggered to his feet. "I'm okay."

The other students started giggling.

Mrs. Offenheimer placed her hands on her hips and glared at Andrea, who turned bright red.

"I'm so sorry," Andrea said. "Bob, Mrs. Offenheimer, I'm so very sorry."

Bob disentangled himself from the sheets and waved his hand as if to say *no problem.*

Mrs. Offenheimer just moved on to the next lesson. "Well, now that you know how to make the bed, it is time to move on to giving a bath."

How difficult could this be? We give ourselves a bath regularly, well, most of us anyway. Except Sally. Oh, how we waited for someone to tell her to take a bath. Our eyes would water, coupled with a sense of nausea, when she came near us.

We didn't get the chore—opportunity?—of giving Sally a bath. Fortunately, we used mannequins as patients. Even so, Cassie and I both got a fit of giggles. I guess you could say we were both a little embarrassed to be talking about body parts. Cassie had long, wavy blonde hair and piercing sky-blue eyes. Her family lived in the burbs, so she stayed in the school dorm.

"Girls, get serious." Mrs. Offenheimer gave us a stern look. We were taking a bit longer than the others.

CHAPTER ONE FIRST YEAR OF NURSING SCHOOL

Next up was the job of transferring a patient from the bed to the chair and vice versa. Cassie asked to be the nurse first, and she followed instructions by dangling me first at the side of the bed to get me acclimated to being upright. From there, she wrapped her arms around my upper trunk and under my armpits to get me into a standing position. From there, she slowly pivoted to turn me and gradually lowered me into the chair.

Then she hopped on the bed. I swung her feet over, grabbed her around the trunk, giggling, and started to pivot. Then I felt something between the floor and me.

I had stepped on Cassie's foot! Luckily my whole weight wasn't on that leg. I looked up at her.

She didn't even flinch.

I lowered her into the chair, grateful that she hadn't shouted or something.

"Good job, girls." Mrs. Offenheimer apparently hadn't noticed my mistake.

Cassie and I shared a smile.

We moved on to ambulating each other. This involved walking alongside our partner with one arm wrapped around the back and the other arm grasping the forearm providing the support. We moved onto the task of supervising ambulation with a cane and a walker.

Cassie was taller than me by about six inches, but I was still able to execute this task without difficulty.

While it may seem elementary, we had to know how to safely use a wheelchair as well, primarily due to the need to properly install leg rests, foot pedals, and locks. You would have thought that some of us had a screw lose in our brains trying to put the pieces together. This task took a long time to complete.

Once Mrs. Offenheimer was satisfied with our wheelchair assembly and operation skills, we moved on to that wonderful job of toileting a bedbound patient with a urinal and a bedpan. We also had to transfer a patient to a bedside commode or traditional toilet. We were expected to complete this task while making it a private and comfortable experience.

This time, I was partnered with Bob.

Initially, I had to give him a urinal. This was the easiest because I just had to hand it to him or place it under the sheet. Next, I had to place Bob on a bedpan while he was in bed. This involves rolling the patient from his or her back to one side while keeping him or her covered.

As you recall, Bob was a large fellow, and I did not want him to fall again.

I yanked on the side rail to check that it was secure. "Not gonna let you fall this time."

When he was on his side, facing away from me, I lifted the sheet just enough to slide the bedpan under his buttocks and rolled him back to the center, so he was facing the ceiling. I raised the head of the bed, putting him in a sitting position. I was perspiring and flushed, I felt a bit embarrassed doing this for a man.

When we finished, Mrs. Offenheimer pulled me aside. "Are you all right or just embarrassed?"

"Just embarrassed." I pulled my chin up. "But I will get past this."

She smiled. "Yes, you will."

Medication administration was another of the most important nursing basics. Knowing the five rights of medication administration was drilled in our heads: the right patient, the right medicine, the right dose, the right route, and the right time.

As we moved onto technical tasks, I needed to move past a fear of blood draws. Since my childhood, I had always felt faint just seeing a tourniquet and a needle.

My fear was tested when we watched a video presentation about performing a blood draw. As I witnessed the tourniquet being wrapped around the upper arm, I felt a sensation of perspiration in my face and hands. As the

CHAPTER ONE FIRST YEAR OF NURSING SCHOOL

image showed the needle brought to the skin to penetrate the blood vessel, my vision faded, and I felt weak.

I had to do something before I made a fool of myself by passing out—just by watching a video!

Get it together, Aubrey. You have to do this. You can get past this. You wanna be a nurse? This is nursing! Get it together. Breathe!

After a few minutes, the feeling passed. Thank heaven!

Hospital Clinical Rotations

Hospital clinical rotations began after the third month at St. Christopher's Hospital. We were expected to complete one day a week of hospital clinical experience during our first year. Our instructors were assigned units and were available to answer our questions and concerns.

Our first endeavors included patients with conditions including diabetes, heart disease, and lung complications. Our instructor for this rotation was Mrs. Tedesco. She was an attractive, well-endowed, average-weight woman who was always smiling. She had short jet-black hair and wore her makeup well. But somehow, I didn't feel I could trust her—you know, when those innate instincts kick in.

Mrs. Tedesco gave us our assignments the day before our instruction began, with all of the necessary particulars. This gave us the opportunity to look up the medical information ahead of time, so we would be prepared and could write a care plan. The care plan is a document outlining the diagnosis, patient assessment, interventions, rationale, and outcome. To further define a care plan, it is a list of the medical ailments, results of a patient's responses to our inquiries on how they feel, our physical examinations, what we did to help them and the results of our care.

On the morning of our initial clinical rotation, we dressed in our uniforms and student caps, which were small and plain compared to those of the licensed nurses. We entered St. Christopher's Hospital via the famous

Nursing, Yes I Do!

tunnel and took the elevator to reach Six East Wing. This tunnel connected the nursing school to St. Christopher's Hospital.

The team leader and some of the staff were not happy to see us.

"Ugh. I hate this," the team leader whispered.

A nurse replied, "Students. What a waste of our time."

Well, there we were, at morning report with a bitch of a team leader. This baffled me. After all, we bathed, dressed, mobilized, toileted, medicated, and performed treatments on their patients.

The team leader was responsible for giving each of us a shift report on our patients, so we knew how they had done during the night shift. She was minimalistic in her reports, leaving many gaps in patient information. For instance, with one patient, she neglected to tell us he was scheduled for a transfer to another hospital which led to mass confusion for the student assigned making her look like an imbecile. As a result, we started reviewing the charts to learn more on our own.

My first patient was a seventy-five-year-old male diagnosed with severe lung disease—secondary to his smoking—and extreme confusion due to dementia.

I entered the room. "Good morning, my name is Aubrey. I'll be taking care of you today."

He had a tabloid in his hands. "Karen, I need you to go place my bets on three horses scheduled to race today."

"Sir, I'm Aubrey, your nurse."

He turned a page of his paper, the *Daily Racing Form*. "No, you are Karen, my assistant. Now get me my clothes, order my car, and place my bets."

I could not successfully reorient him. He grew angry, rolling up the newspaper and waving it like a club.

How am I gonna get out of this? "I need to take care of something first. I'll be back soon." I left the room and sped down the hall to the head nurse's station.

CHAPTER ONE FIRST YEAR OF NURSING SCHOOL

Fortunately, she was much nicer than some of the other staff. She chuckled. "Go back in a few minutes with his medications. I'm sure he will have totally forgotten what he said."

And she was right.

Cassie's patient was a seventy-year-old male down the hall. He had chronic diarrhea as well as episodic hallucinations.

Cassie noticed a horrible stench when she walked in the room, and after introducing herself, she realized he was sitting in a small lake of liquid stool. "Sir, are you all right?"

"Oh, I love laying on the wet sand and taking in the sunshine." He thought he was sitting on the beach.

Cassie gasped and ran out of the room.

In the corridor, she grabbed me. "I need help."

The head nurse was in earshot and asked what had happened. She calmed Cassie and gathered a couple of nurse aides, plenty of towels, and clean linens to assist with the cleanup.

Just as we practiced in class, we rolled the patient and cleaned him up. At least the patient was compliant.

When we finished and got him settled comfortably, he asked, "When can I go back to the beach?"

My other patient was a seventy-five-year-old gentleman with a severe heart condition known as congestive heart failure. He also had poor bladder control related to his benign prostatic hypertrophy (BPH, or what we would now call benign prostatic hyperplasia: an enlargement of the prostate gland.)

He weighed about three hundred pounds and was non-ambulatory, meaning he couldn't walk on his own. I needed help to re-position him in bed and change his diaper. He was alert and oriented and very embarrassed about his dependencies. He thanked me frequently during my shift. I bathed, dressed, toileted, and transferred him out of bed with help, and then I medicated him.

By the end of the shift, I was exhausted—not in body but in mind. My mental fatigue was likely the product of my level of anxiety since this was my first day on clinical rotations. At any rate, I met the expected goals for treatment, and my patient was satisfied with his care.

Afterward, we were responsible for preparing a patient summary: a thorough description of the patient, care provided, and the patient's response.

I completed my first patient summary and handed it in to Mrs. Tedesco.

She gave me a failing grade.

No one at the hospital had criticized my work, so I was very confused.

After class I approached her. "Mrs. Tedesco, can you explain why I got this grade?"

She huffed as if I were intruding, and she had little advice for me.

Before I walked home, I met some girls at the dorm for study group. It was easier for us to meet there since I was the only one commuting. The others were all on campus. Corrine led the study group. She would pick the topic of the day, whether it be the heart, lungs, muscles, etcetera. She would toss out questions to each of us to reinforce what we learned.

We gathered around a table in the common room of the dorm, and I showed my paper to Corrine, Cassie, Penny, Missy, and Rhonda. They all pulled out their papers too.

Cassie had received a grade of ninety-five.

"Let me see that." Corrine compared Cassie's paper with mine to see what I was lacking. Corrine was always the go-to person for questions about what we covered in class. She could present any topic clearly. "The only difference I can see," Corrine said, "is that Cassie's handwriting is schoolbook perfect and yours... isn't."

I couldn't deny it. I hadn't expected to be graded on penmanship.

The girls agreed that I had fulfilled all the guidelines for the paper and felt I deserved at least a passing grade.

Labs and Classes

Our curriculum included anatomy and physiology, which was taught by Ms. Simple. She had an amazing smile and managed to keep our class completely engaged.

I found the class intriguing—I enjoyed getting to know the parts of the body and how they worked. The laboratory portion was another story.

In the lab we dissected insects, cats, and brains—just to mention a few subjects. The tissues were preserved in formaldehyde, which, although colorless, smells like musty pickles.

Initially, the smell was nauseating, but eventually we became nose blind.

One day, I surprised my mother by bringing home a cat brain to study. Yes, it was contained in a jar filled with formaldehyde. And it was ugly.

Upon seeing that jar in my hands, Mom almost passed out.

Anatomy lab was on Wednesday mornings, so to avoid any disruption to my stomach, I had to avoid consuming too much at the local drinking establishment on Tuesday nights.

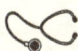

General Psychology was my favorite class, taught by Ms. Smith, a fiftyish woman with short blonde hair who dressed casually. She did an excellent job of presenting the topic.

The day I took my first exam, I was running a fever of 102 degrees. On that day, our area was hit by an ice storm. Since I was not feeling well, my father picked me up from school.

As we drove home, I noticed something unusual I had never seen before. Icicles hanging from tree branches looked like Christmas trees minus the green. With my high fever, I was not sure if I was hallucinating or if it was real.

Either way, I got a grade of ninety-nine on the test, and finished the class with a final grade of A+, so I couldn't have been too ill.

Per my request, Mrs. Appleworth became my personal clinical advisor instead of Mrs. Tedesco after the penmanship incident. She was wonderful. Twelve of us were in her group, and like a homeroom teacher, she would sometimes hug those of us who were right out of high school because she knew that we got scared. She took time to sit with us and was empathetic because she had entered nursing school right out of high school.

She had red hair, glasses, and an average build. She stuttered at times and was occasionally forgetful. We appreciated her kindness and approachability, so we overlooked the flaws that, if we were still in high school, we might have teased her for.

Mrs. Appleworth was responsible for compiling grades for the students in her group and held occasional meetings with us to help alleviate our fears and avoid unnecessary failures. "As you get older and gain experience," she said, "the work will be much easier, and you won't need hugs—except in extreme situations."

Her advice was that nursing is a job dealing directly with human life, therefore we would be inhumane if we totally withheld emotion, but she explained that we should choose our times for displaying that emotion wisely, so as not to cloud our judgment. She warned us that if we developed

CHAPTER ONE FIRST YEAR OF NURSING SCHOOL

a personal liking or disliking for a patient, our decision making would be based on personal feelings as opposed to our education and clinical experience. As a result, the patient's outcome would suffer.

With my subsequent patient summaries graded by Mrs. Appleworth, along with my classroom participation, quizzes, and tests, I was able to raise my cumulative grade to an A minus. I despised the paperwork but enjoyed the patient care. Each time the instructors taught a new technique, I was fearful but eager to learn.

Code Blue

On my first rotation to the gastrointestinal unit, I cared for Lorelei, a female patient who was fifty years old and suffered with esophageal varices (enlarged veins) and cirrhosis of the liver, secondary to a thirty-year history of excessive drinking.

One the second day of my assignment with her, I finished changing her bed and grabbed her chart to refresh my memory about her treatment plan.

"Thank you, Aubrey. You're really helpful."

"You're welcome. That's why I'm here."

She plucked at her blanket. "I know I'm only sick because of the drinking. But . . . can I tell you something?"

She sounded so serious. I put the chart down and returned to her bedside. "Sure."

"The drinking, it's just . . . how I cope, y'know. Life's been hard." Her voice cracked.

"I understand."

"I bet you don't!" Lorelei sounded angry. "My stepfather sexually abused me, beginning when I was only seven, up to my seventeenth birthday."

What could I say to that? I had no words.

"I finally built up the courage to tell my mother about it, but she didn't believe me. I felt ashamed and all alone and decided to run away from home."

I pulled up a chair. If she needed to talk, I could listen.

"I met this other girl on the street. She was eighteen. She let me stay with her. We became good friends. I found solace there. And she taught me how to turn tricks for money. The apartment was small, and we ate little food, but we drank hard alcohol, like, daily." Lorelei cast her eyes toward the ceiling. "Oddly, I developed kind of a . . . a sense of control with the men, and comfort from the alcohol. That helped mask the pain of the . . . abuse." She began to sob.

I handed her a couple tissues and held her hand until she was ready to talk again.

"When I turned twenty, I stopped turning tricks. I found a job waitressing and an apartment of my own. But I could not stop the drinking . . . 'cause it numbed the pain. After about two years, I met an amazing man." Her voice softened. "He was loving and caring. We married after dating only six months. We had two beautiful children together; one girl and one boy. I hid the secret and pain of the abuse from him and my children. Somehow, I successfully hid my daily drinking, until about two years ago. When my husband challenged me about it, I decided it was time to tell him and the kids about the sexual abuse. I was shocked but relieved by their response. They hugged me and cried with me for hours. My husband recommended counseling, which I promptly began. It was extremely helpful."

Her voice was a little stronger now. "Unfortunately, I started having pain in my belly. Dizziness. Blood in my stool. My doctor started treatments, but I only got worse. And here I am." She patted my hand. "Thank you, Aubrey, for listening to me. I needed to get that out." Lorelei began to cry again.

I sat next to her on the bed and held her tightly for a minute.

CHAPTER ONE FIRST YEAR OF NURSING SCHOOL

Then she patted my shoulder and pulled away. "I am very tired and would like to go to sleep."

With that said, I left the room to let her rest.

Later in my shift, Lorelei began to bleed from her rectum. I notified the charge nurse and sought help from my fellow students who had worked as aides before entering nursing school. They taught me how to master cleaning her backside with a bath towel by rolling it over and over to use every part of the towel to wipe her.

After one hour and three episodes of rectal bleeding, she then began to bleed from her nose and mouth. I summoned the charge nurse again, who, after witnessing the bleeding, called the in-house medical resident.

The resident listened to Lorelei's heart. "She's fibrillating." This is a condition in which the chambers of the heart no longer beat in sync.

The charge nurse pressed the button in the room labeled "Code Blue." This summoned a team of medical staff to resuscitate Lorelei. Each hospital may have their own name but here, it is written as "Code Blue." This indicates the need for lifesaving measures for a patient or any individual at that location. It has been known to be used for a family member or even a staff member. A button is present in every patient room and when pressed, it triggers the hospital receptionist to make an announcement over the intercom such as Code Blue, followed by the name of the unit. This in turn triggers all of the members of the code team in the hospital to respond and treat the affected individual. The code team includes one or more physicians, one or more critical care nurses and a respiratory therapist. When the team arrives, the existing staff of the unit will assist the team.

It all happened so fast. Within thirty minutes, she fell into a coma. We put in an endotracheal tube and respirator—this forces air into the lungs. We tried intravenous fluids and medications to revive her organ and vascular function. And we defibrillated—delivering an electrical shock to the heart to try to reestablish a normal heart rhythm.

All our efforts proved to no avail. Time of death was 2:05 p.m.

Mrs. Appleworth took my hand and led me to the nurses' lounge. There we sat down, and I wept and muttered. "She told me her whole life story...as if she had to get it out before . . ." I couldn't say any more.

She apparently knew exactly how I felt and hugged me. "You are in shock right now, and that's what is giving you that weird uneasy and numb sensation."

How did she know exactly what I was feeling? I guessed she'd been there.

"But it will pass," she continued. "The first loss is the worst. You will learn to handle it better as time goes on. You'll learn to compartmentalize your feelings so you can continue working and take care of your other patients."

Chapter Two

SECOND YEAR OF NURSING SCHOOL

Sister Roach's voice droned at the edges of my consciousness. I just needed to close my eyes for a second...

Someone nudged my arm. Penny. I smiled my thanks, and she nodded as if to say, "You're welcome." I'd done the same favor for her in the past.

Sister Roach was a kind and caring instructor, but her class, Religious Philosophy, was a sleeper. No disrespect to our Lord intended, but it was the last class of the day. And since Christolette was a Catholic college, it was required. So, we sleepy students looked out for each other.

Nursing school grew increasingly complex, with added academics like microbiology—the study of the human cell and how it affects our general health. Class work included studying diseases of all body systems that filled a book I could barely wrap my arms around. Our clinical time at St. Christopher's increased to two days per week, however with our experience, the work became a little easier.

Orthopedics

My next assignment was an orthopedic rotation. Orthopedics is the field of medicine involving the study of muscles and bones. Our lead instructor, Mrs. Offenheimer, kept us on our toes to make sure we maintained a good schedule of monitoring strength and tone of the muscles and proper alignment of limbs of our patients. We also maintained supportive devices such as splints, weights, and recommended traction devices.

Since most of these patients had limited mobility, we had to frequently reposition them to prevent bed sores. But even using good body mechanics ourselves, we felt the aches and pains the next day. Tylenol became our best friend.

Surgery

We moved on to the surgical unit and here again, I was assigned to work with Mrs. Tedesco. I decided to use a different approach to her by presenting myself with more self-confidence, and that worked well.

The surgical rotation was extremely busy in the early morning as we got everyone ready for their surgeries. No time here to make small talk with your patient.

Now it was time to run through the surgical pre-op checklist:
- Consent signed
- Labs done
- History, physical and consult in chart
- Pre-op injection given
- Jewelry removed
- Make-up removed
- Surgical site shave/prep done

If the surgery involved the need to shave the "private areas," a staff member of the same gender routinely completed this task—except in emergency cases.

My patient was a sixty-year-old male awaiting a hiatal hernia repair. I completed the pre-op check list, and he was ready to go. Mrs. Tedesco stood by, ready to sign me off on any tasks I completed, beginning with my first intramuscular injection on a live patient.

CHAPTER TWO SECOND YEAR OF NURSING SCHOOL

In the medicine room, I took out two syringes to draw up the ordered medications. My hands shook, and I felt a sharp pain in my finger. I had accidentally stuck myself. This is pretty common among health care workers. Since this needle was clean, the only problem was that I had contaminated it.

Mrs. Tedesco frowned and sighed with exasperation.

A staff nurse leaned on the doorframe, impatiently waiting for me to finish so she could use the medicine room.

My intention to show self-confidence shattered. My hands shook even worse as I pinched my finger to stop the bleeding.

Mrs. Tedesco turned to the staff nurse. "Please give us a couple extra minutes."

The nurse furrowed her brow.

Before she could speak, Mrs. Tedesco added, "Do you remember when you were preparing your first intramuscular injection as a nursing student?"

The nurse blushed, ducked her head, and walked away.

"Start over," Mrs. Tedesco's voice was firm but not unkind.

I took out another needle, picked up the medicine vial, double-checked the dosage, and filled the syringes.

Next, I placed the two filled syringes of medicine on a tray with the med cards and entered my patient's room, with Mrs. Tedesco close behind. I explained the shots and asked him to roll over. He smiled and obliged my request.

After I had given him the injections, Mrs. Tedesco nodded her approval.

My patient rolled over and sat up. "First time, huh?"

"Yes, how did I do?"

"Best shot I ever received."

We all laughed, and my anxiety vanished.

Next we were invited to observe in the operating room. The surgery scheduled was a repair of a right fractured hip.

Mrs. Tedesco showed us where to stand. "Stay out of the way, and once you're in your spot, do not move."

I stood to one side of the patient, behind the surgical team but with enough room to see what was going on. My classmate Jenny stood at the head of the operating table.

About ten minutes into the procedure, Jenny slowly leaned to one side and gracefully tipped over onto the floor. Passed out cold.

We wanted to help her, but we were frozen in our spots by Mrs. Tedesco's command.

The surgeon looked up and pointed to one of the techs. "Check on her and move her out of the way."

I was a little pleased with myself for not having passed out in the operating room.

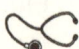

After that, I had the opportunity to witness a circumcision. I came in after they'd started and before I could stop myself, blurted "Oh my God!"

There were more metal devices than baby. As I got closer and looked into his eyes, they were swollen and red. The rest of his little body was a burgundy red, and he was crying profusely. The metal device attached to his little penis was anchored securely, and blood from the circumcision leaked out.

Before I knew it, I felt woozy, and all the blood drained from my face.

The physician glared at me. "Go sit down and put your head between your knees."

I did this promptly.

Afterward, the physician sat down beside me. "You okay?"

"Yes, thank you." I rubbed my forehead. "I am sorry."

CHAPTER TWO SECOND YEAR OF NURSING SCHOOL

"No problem. Happens all the time."

What a day. That night, I was glad to get home and into bed.

Obstetrics and Gynecology

It was now time to move forward with my obstetrics and gynecology (also known as OB/GYN). Obstetrics is the field of medicine involving the care of a female during and after pregnancy. Gynecology is the field of medicine of the health and well-being of the female productive system. As a woman, I was certainly interested in what was involved in having a baby.

Mrs. Sanborn, a white-haired lady about sixty years old, taught the OB/GYN courses. She was profoundly serious, and rarely showed emotion.

Which isn't to say she *never* showed emotion.

One day as I worked on charts, Mrs. Sanborn ran over to me. "Your mother just called. She said a man called her and said he had taken you away."

I just stared, perplexed. "What? Why?"

"Who knows? Prankster maybe. But your mother is concerned. You had better call her back right away."

I called my mother, who was indeed a bit frantic, and let her know I was fine. We never found out who made this call and never received another one of this nature.

I found this level of concern for someone who wasn't a patient reassuring because this was not Mrs. Sanborn's usual personality.

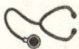

My first obstetric patient—I'll call her Erica—was a twenty-five-year-old first-time mother. She arrived in the labor department at 9 a.m. with irregular contractions.

I observed while the labor nurse examined the patient. The nurse explained to the patient—and me—the labor process, involving the dilation and thinning of the cervix, the opening at the bottom of the uterus.

Nursing, Yes I Do!

The labor nurse made notes on the patient's chart. "At the moment, you're not in active labor—"

"How is that possible?" Erica's voice verged on panic.

The labor nurse nodded as if she understood the shock. "Our definition of 'active' is based on the condition of your cervix and the timing of your contractions." She put the chart away. "I recommend you take a walk in the hall. Aubrey will accompany you."

Erica sighed. "All right."

As she and I walked up and down the hall, we became wrapped in conversation.

"I never expected to have a baby," she said.

"Why not?"

"When I was fourteen, the obstetrician said I had a 'juvenile uterus,' so I would most likely never have children." I knew that juvenile uterus is a condition in which the uterus is smaller than normal. My patient continued, "And if I did, I'd need a C-section to deliver the baby."

"I can relate. I had a similar experience with my first OB/GYN."

"Yeah. I was scared because I wanted to have children. So, I didn't go back to him." We reached the end of the hall and turned around to go the other way.

"Did you talk to another obstetrician?"

She laughed a little. "Not until six months ago."

"And what did they say?"

"They told me my pregnancy was progressing as expected. But, that fear . . ." Her voice dropped. "It's still in the back of my mind."

I paused at the door of Erica's room. "Do you want to keep going?"

"Nah, I'd rather lie down now."

I settled her in her room and left her alone to rest.

Within two hours, my patient's cervix showed readiness for delivery, and her contractions were coming approximately every two minutes.

CHAPTER TWO SECOND YEAR OF NURSING SCHOOL

I followed Erica to the delivery room with the baby's father, the physician, and the nursing staff. Since she was fully dilated and effaced, it was safe to push, so this was encouraged.

I never realized the contortion of agony on a woman's face during delivery of a baby. My mind wandered. *I may not want to do this myself.*

The obstetrician delivered the baby vaginally—perfectly safely—and cut the cord. I heard the baby's first cry, and my heart melted at seeing a new life brought into this world.

A labor nurse brought the baby to the mother's bare chest, and I watched in awe as she and her husband stroked and kissed their newborn child. Erica and I shared a blink and a head nod. Her fear of a C-section was history.

Yes, I want children too.

For my gynecology rotation, I was assigned a high-priority patient after she refused to have one of my male colleague's care for her. She was a highly respected local journalist.

When I went in to provide her morning bed bath, I noticed her hesitance to disrobe. So, I gave her the utmost privacy. Following her bath, I felt a sense of increased trust.

She readjusted her pajamas. "I'm sorry, I don't mean to be snippy. I just—I'm so frightened." Her steely demeanor broke, and she wept. "I used to be so independent and now—cancer! I don't know what I'm going to do. I feel so helpless."

I listened intently as she sobbed between her words. The loss of her independent life devastated her, and she welcomed my embrace to comfort her while she wept.

Pediatrics

Mrs. Jones was our pediatric instructor. She was the vision of a young grandmother, with prematurely gray hair, glasses, and an open-door policy. She often used humor in her presentations, and her high-pitched voice made them even more hilarious. Her daughter was one of the nursing students in our class, and her voice was the same. We loved them both dearly.

The children on the pediatric floor ranged from six months to sixteen years old.

I was assigned to a four-year-old girl, Bailey. She had cystic fibrosis and had gone into a respiratory exacerbation. Cystic fibrosis is a genetic disorder involving the lungs, digestive system, and other organs. Cells affected by the disease produce abnormal mucus, sweat, and digestive juices. These fluids become sticky and thick, causing the tubes, ducts, and other passageways to become clogged. This causes shortness of breath in the lungs.

Respiratory exacerbation is a flare up of symptoms in which the patient's cough and shortness of breath become worse. Bailey needed to be in a misted tent and receive nebulizer treatments to keep her air passages open. The nebulizer converts medicine to a mist so it can be breathed into the lungs to treat the air passageways.

When I entered the room, Bailey's eyes just gazed at me, and I softly spoke to her.

"Bailey, my name is Aubrey, and I am here to help you feel better today."

She raised her arms to be picked up.

I had been told she could be out of the tent briefly, so I took the opportunity to let her out, hoping that would help her feel comfortable with me. It felt nice to hold this little darling in my arms, but I had only a few minutes.

I grabbed a picture book from the bedside stand, sat in the rocking chair, and went through a couple of pages in the book. I brought her attention back to me and then returned her to the crib without stopping my conversation. "This is a magical bed. It will give you medicine to help you feel better."

This was a good day, and I thought I might like working in a pediatric unit.

Private Lives

One Friday, after my morning class, I sat in the lounge. We were all pretty relaxed that day, looking forward to the weekend. One of my nursing classmates, Rosanne, sat nearby. She had a 4.0 average, but I could never figure out how she had such good grades, because she always appeared to be high on something or other.

"Hello, how are you doing?" I said.

She replied, "You will never guess what happened to me last weekend."

"Something good, I hope."

"No, not good. I was hanging out with friends at Mullens, having a few drinks, and then went next door to the Eagle's Nest for more drinks. I went in the bathroom, and someone must have put something in my drink, because the next thing I knew, I was in the ICU (Intensive Care Unit) on a ventilator."

I gasped. "Oh, my God! You're apparently okay now. Do you know what was in your drink?"

She shook her head.

"Well... I'm glad you're all right now." I did not believe all of what she said. In the back of my mind, I thought, *Sure... someone else drugged you.*

Nights at Hoppin' Joe's

Despite all this hard work, I found time to relax. When I started nursing school, I was dating a boy named Clark. He was handsome, but he thought way too much of himself. Our relationship lasted about three months.

Nursing, Yes I Do!

After Clark, I dated Ken for about four months. I had known Ken in high school, but we had never dated then. Ken stood five feet, eight inches tall, with an average build. He was nice looking and home on leave from the navy. We had fun together, but the spark was not there for me. He wanted to get engaged; I had to use my best tactics to let him down easily, because I hated to hurt anyone's feelings.

While I was dating Ken, a high school friend named Kelly called about going together to Hoppin' Joe's on Tuesday nights for drinks and dancing. The drinks were fifty percent off, which was great on my tight budget. My mother taught me to watch my spending.

Hoppin' Joe's was a huge place with a dance floor set up like a runway for models and lit up with colored lights that shifted with the music.

On one particular Tuesday, Kelly, Ken, and I headed to Hoppin' Joe's. When we arrived, I noticed a very handsome guy exiting a car nearby.

Kelly shouted, "Hey Ethan!"

The guy turned around and waved in our direction.

I felt that spark I had been waiting for, like fireworks in my brain. I never felt that with Ken.

Ken took my hand—which was suddenly very warm—and we headed inside.

After Ken and I had a couple of dances and a drink, Ethan walked over. He looked at Ken. "Hi. May I have a dance with the lady?"

Ken looked at me.

"He's a friend of Kelly's. I'll be right back."

Ken just nodded.

I walked with Ethan to the dance floor. I noticed a girl in the vicinity of where he had come from looking directly at me. *He must be on the outs with his date.* Since my date was headed back to the navy, I thought this would all turn out okay.

CHAPTER TWO SECOND YEAR OF NURSING SCHOOL

It was a fast dance. The Bump was a popular dance move at that time, so it became part of our dance for that song.

The song ended. We exchanged smiles and Ethan walked me off the floor.

I headed back to Ken. Ken and I had a delightful evening and danced together for a couple of slow songs. But even before Ethan turned up, Ken knew this might be our last outing based on the discouraging look on his face when he bid me farewell as he left to return to his role in the navy.

The next time I saw Ethan at Hoppin' Joe's, we were both unattached. I rode with three other girls I knew from high school. I was only close to one of the girls. The other two were just no more than acquaintances. Unbeknownst to me, one of the girls was an old girlfriend of Ethan's. Her name was Polly. Upon entering Hoppin Joes, my eyes were searching for Ethan and within seconds, his eyes met mine and we quickly moved towards each other and grasped hands. We danced and had a great time; however, an awkward moment followed. When Polly saw us together, she went up to Ethan and slapped him in the face. My jaw dropped at the site of this. Ethan asked for privacy to speak to her. I walked away but kept an eye on the two of them from a distance. I could tell there were words being said by the two of them. Ethan appeared calm and in control while she was visibly upset and eventually walked away. Ethan came up to me, apologized and said that he broke it off with her two months ago because she was suffocating him. We continued to have an enjoyable evening but hearing that, I had no intention of asking him for a ride home as this might look like I was desperate, so I rode home in the same car I arrived in including his ex-girlfriend. She cried intermittently during our whole trip. I thought it was best to just keep quiet during the car ride but said I am sorry if I hurt you as I exited the car. This was one of my worst experiences.

Psychiatric Rotation

During our last semester, we had to complete a rotation at the BAS Psychiatric Institute. On the day of our assignment, I carpooled with my classmate Linda, but we left our homes late, and I tried to make up the time by driving fast. I had no problem finding the place; we could see its palatial spires from the road. We arrived about ten minutes late and nervously hurried into the building and to the receptionist.

I was short of breath when I spoke. "We're nursing students in Mr. Morris's class. Can you direct us to where he's meeting with our class?"

She didn't even look up. "Sorry, but he's not here today."

Linda handed her a copy of our schedule. "Please check again."

"All right, I guess I'll have him paged."

The public address system must have been in some back office because the receptionist disappeared through a door.

In the interim. Linda and I grew increasingly nervous since we were not yet comfortable dealing with the mentally ill as this was our first live experience. Our studies have shown that the mentally ill often have behavior issues and fear being on the wrong side of a situation. Our trepidation increased when an exceptionally large man approached us. He must have stood seven feet tall and three feet wide. He did not say a word but bent and extended his hand. We each shook his hand. Then, he just turned and walked away without a word.

While he did not hurt us, we exchanged a look of terror.

Finally, the receptionist returned. "Your class is on the third floor. You can take the stairs on your right."

We grabbed each other's hand and walked toward the stairwell and up to the third floor. After ducking down some hallways, we found Mr. Morris and the class in the conference room and apologized for our tardiness.

CHAPTER TWO SECOND YEAR OF NURSING SCHOOL

Mr. Morris was very understanding. We sat down, and before Mr. Morris could speak further, a patient walked into the conference room with his pants unzipped, showing a shadow of his penis, and holding three cigarettes in his mouth.

"Roy, please zip up your pants and leave the room," Mr. Morris said gently but firmly. "I am teaching a class."

The patient complied.

I listened more intently to Mr. Morris than I had ever listened to a teacher before. He gave us examples of the types of mental illnesses treated at this facility and what he expected of us to complete a work assignment. In short, we were to develop a rapport with a patient using therapeutic communication and draft a report using the steps provided to us in class.

"Use caution around a patient who appears volatile," he said, "and find me or a staff member as needed."

On my way down the hall, I found a young man who reminded me of a high school classmate, which gave me shivers as I remembered him as being somewhat of a recluse. I approached him. "Would you like to talk?"

He had six cigarettes hanging out of his mouth and responded with a grunt.

"It's okay; maybe another time." I walked away.

One of my female classmates, Betty, sat at a table in the community room speaking to another patient. Betty had worked as an aide before attending the nursing program. She was a beauty. Her eyes, nose, and mouth were so perfectly shaped and placed on her face; it was like looking at Whitney Houston. Her long, dark hair lay gently on her shoulders, and her figure was Barbie-doll perfect.

"Betty, do you mind if I sit in?"

She smiled. "Sure."

The patient was a tall, slender black man with a rugged, unkempt beard.

Fortunately, Betty had not started her interview yet. Looking straight into the patient's eyes, she identified herself and me. "As students in the nursing program, we're here to learn about your condition and the care you receive here."

He rose to his feet. "I am George Washington Carver." He sat back down and looked intently into Betty's eyes. "Boy, you have sexy lips." He followed this non sequitur with statements that were quite normal, speaking about his childhood. About every three minutes thereafter, for the fifteen minutes I sat there, he repeated the sequence of the *George Washington Carver* and *boy, you have sexy lips* thing.

At that point, I excused myself to find a patient of my own. On my way into the hall, one of the female staff members grabbed me and pulled me into a nurses' station with three other people, and the door was locked behind us.

Through a window in the door, we saw a young man run past, yelling, and flailing his arms. He continued to run up and down the hall, in uncontrolled emotional chaos.

After about ten minutes without another appearance, we called the front desk and were advised that it was safe to leave the room.

I timidly walked to one of the common rooms and found a man in a red jacket with an industry emblem embroidered on it. He stood about six feet tall, was a little overweight, and had unkempt blond hair and brown eyes.

I began with an approach similar to Betty's. I introduced myself as a nursing student and asked if I could speak to him for a bit.

He looked down at me inquisitively but agreed.

I was immediately impressed with his ability to initiate the conversation about himself and his work advancing televisions. He answered my questions appropriately, and I was ecstatic. I had all the information I needed for my paper.

CHAPTER TWO SECOND YEAR OF NURSING SCHOOL

When I left the room, I sought out a staff member and asked, "Why is this man here? He seems so normal."

She looked over her glasses at me.

My stomach knotted. I realized I had really demonstrated my inexperience with mentally ill people.

The staff member took off her glasses and drew a deep breath. "He raped his mother and threw her down the basement stairs to her death."

I immediately got shivers all the way down my spine.

Linda and I talked about our crazy experiences all the way home. We both decided psychiatric nursing was not for us.

Graduation

After my two years of study and hard work, graduation time arrived. But before that, we had our capping and pinning ceremony. It's worth noting that the boys did not require a cap . . . sexist, huh?

We each had a new, crisp white uniform for the ceremony, which was held at Bastille's Music Hall. The place brought back memories. The last time I had been there was five years earlier, performing in a dance recital. The unique venue was shaped like a drum, with a concert hall inside, where the philharmonic performed, and a smaller room for events like our ceremony.

We were all more excited about this event than our graduation. We were officially nurses . . . that is, assuming we would pass our state boards.

My parents, sister, and now boyfriend, Ethan, accompanied me to the ceremony. My sixty classmates and I lined up neatly, waiting to cross the auditorium stage to receive our caps and pins.

My heart raced. My name was called, and I walked onto the stage. I felt myself glowing as I received my cap. The caps may have been starchy and old fashioned, but they weren't just symbols of the school, they represented all the hard work we had put into success.

Nursing, Yes I Do!

It was a beautiful warm spring day in May, and we made the most of it by ending with a celebratory dinner at Passucci's.

I do not want to slight graduation, as it was the following month at the same venue. At that event, we wore traditional white gowns and mortarboard caps to receive our Associate of Science in Nursing (ASN) degrees.

I recall just feeling relieved. No more school—at least for a while.

Chapter Three

MOVING FORWARD AFTER SCHOOL

With school completed, I enjoyed more free time with Ethan. When we dated for a year, he popped that magical question... in his own way.

"What would you say if I asked you to marry me?"

I said yes.

We found the perfect ring and set a date for April 28 of the following year. We had so much to do—looking for a dress, flowers, cake, church, and reception hall. I decided on six attendants and one flower girl.

Preparing for the Future

Not only was I preparing for my wedding, but I was also studying for my nursing state board exam to ultimately receive my nursing license. They were scheduled for three months after graduation, and this did not prevent us from working. A nurse was allowed to work as a Graduate Nurse (GN) for about eighteen months, as I recall, before passing the state board exams.

Cassie, Corrine, Penny, Rhonda, Missy, and I were to take the exams in Niagara Falls in the autumn. The exams were scheduled over two days, so we made reservations to stay at the Holiday Inn.

In the meantime, I pounded the pavement, dropping off my resume at various local hospitals.

Nursing, Yes I Do!

I have never been one to sit around and waste time, so I was also considering going back to school for my Baccalaureate of Science in Nursing (BSN) because a little birdie in my head said, *You would be better off with your four-year degree.*

Many people told me that if I were offered a job as a GN, it would be an evening shift, so I signed up for day classes to begin in the fall.

Two months went by before I received a call from the Bastille (BAS) Pediatric Center. I gladly went to the interview. I met with the director of nursing, a very attractive woman with dark eyes and hair, high cheekbones, and wearing a burgundy suit. She offered me a full-time position in the intensive care nursery on day shift.

"I'm continuing my studies for my BSN by taking day classes." I thought I was being so professional when I told her this, but it backfired.

Her expression was stern. "I see."

What was I thinking? I just lost out on a great opportunity.

She closed the folder with my resume in it. "Congratulations on your dedication to your studies." She stood. "I'll let you know if we have any openings on the evening shift." She put out her hand, and I shook it.

I left there deflated. The next week, I canceled my registration for BSN studies.

A few days later, I received a call from the Bastille County Hospital (BCH) to set up an interview. As I drove to BCH for my interview, I noticed the neighborhood was run down, with boarded-up shop fronts and graffiti everywhere. I parked the car and walked into the facility, glancing around to make sure I was safe.

Inside, I asked for directions to the office of the director of nurses and was told it was on the second floor. When I reached the office, a shapely, well-endowed female who was dressed to advertise her body contours summoned me and directed me to another room down the hall.

CHAPTER THREE MOVING FORWARD AFTER SCHOOL

There I sat in front of a middle-aged, slender woman with short blonde hair. She wore heavy makeup with bright red lipstick and wore a fully starched white nursing uniform and cap. "I'm Mrs. Spacha." Her sharp, firm demeanor frightened me a bit, but I took care not to let it show.

Apparently, I answered her questions appropriately and revealed myself to be a fit candidate for the job, because she offered me a full-time evening position on the medical/surgical floor.

My starting salary was $5.05 per hour, for a gross of $10,504 per year, which was a good salary for the time. I replied with a "yes" and "thank you" and was asked to meet with her secretary regarding the paperwork. My starting date would be in seven days.

I left there feeling excited but nervous and called my mother to tell her the good news.

It took six rings before my mom answered the phone.

"Mom, I was hired by BCH, and I start next week."

"Oh, I am so happy for you. Tell me more when you get home."

"Absolutely!"

I had to tell Cassie, so I called her too. I was talking so fast and loudly, she had to yell at me.

"Aubrey, stop! Listen! I was hired there too."

"No! What shift?"

"Second shift."

"Ah! And when do you start training?"

She had been given the same training date as I had been given! We planned to drive in together for orientation.

Orientation at First Job

Cassie and I arrived at BCH on a warm, sunny September day, each in a newly purchased uniform and carrying our nurse's cap in a tote so as not to crush it.

Nursing, Yes I Do!

As we entered the building, two men in uniform approached us.

The first was a fellow with jet black hair, dark eyes, and an olive complexion, who stood more than half a head taller than me. "I'm Sal." He took my right hand, kissed it gently and glared into my eyes.

He gestured to his partner. "This is Joe. Welcome to Bastille County Hospital."

Joe was slightly taller than Sal, with brown hair, blue eyes, and a light complexion. Joe then took Cassie's right hand, kissed it and glared into her eyes.

"We're ambulance attendants. We're gonna take you on a tour of the place."

The building had only five floors and about 150 beds. We started on the main floor and viewed the emergency room. We met the head nurse, Meredith Hallorey. She was about ten years older than I and had a slightly round figure, dark long hair, blue eyes, light skin, and a beautiful smile. She demonstrated full control in her department.

"You better get used to the type of patients that come in here and be strong." She made a note on a file and dropped it into a basket. "We get all kinds here: pimps, prostitutes, drug dealers, addicts."

Cassie and I both gasped, but hopefully not too loudly.

Meredith's eyes darted down the hall to a nun who was approaching us, her skirts barely rustling as she walked. "Oh, there's Sister Castille. You should meet her. She works closely with me, and she often goes on runs with these guys." She nodded toward Sal and Joe.

Sal chuckled. "Yeah, she's not your usual nun. A real pistol."

Sister Castille moved fast. "I heard that, Salvatore." She stopped by the nurses' station, and Joe introduced us. "I do love the action of the emergency room," the sister said. "I would never work on the fourth floor . . . much too boring."

CHAPTER THREE MOVING FORWARD AFTER SCHOOL

We had not yet had the pleasure of the fourth floor, but that was a heads up.

Sal rubbed his hands together. "Next stop—cafeteria."

Joe rolled his eyes. "Oh brother. He's gonna tell that story again."

Well, *that* piqued my curiosity.

The small cafeteria held maybe thirty people.

Sal pointed to the window at the edge of the room. "See that hole in the glass?"

I noticed a cone-shaped hole in the thick glass.

"That's from a gunshot, fired by a man with an assault weapon from the roof next door." Sal dashed to the window and pointed to the opposite building. "A Fed sniper with a rifle sat on the roof of the apartment building next door. He was tracking a drug dealer. People said he was responsible for the deaths of some young people. Anyway, over there"— Sal pointed to a different part of the roof— "was this other guy leaning over the edge with *his* rifle."

The suspected drug dealer had been sitting in the cafeteria at the time, sipping a soft drink. The Fed sniper had not known another man was at the opposite edge of the roof. While both men carried deadly weapons, the other man—not the Federal agent—shot first at the man in the cafeteria, killing him instantly.

"But why?" Cassie wailed. "Who was he?"

Sal shrugged. "Dunno. The Feds chased him but didn't catch him. Probably another dealer. Point is—he pointed to a chair, to the window, and back again— "be careful where you sit and check out the windows first."

We stood there for a second, stunned. Sal looked like he was having too much fun. I was convinced his story was sensationalized, but it scared me, just the same.

Joe had remained in the doorway, looking bored. "Can we go now? There's still a lot to cover."

"Yeah, yeah. You ladies mind taking the stairs?"

Joe led us up the stairs to the second floor intensive care unit, which had only four beds. The head nurse was on the phone, so there were no introductions there.

On the east side of the hall was the burn treatment center, where we had to get buzzed in. As we entered, the smell of burned flesh overwhelmed us.

Joe introduced us to Laura Dee, the charge nurse. This unit also had its own supervisor because burn patients would bypass the emergency room and were brought directly to the burn unit.

On the west side of the floor, Joe pointed out the surgical suites. "We can't take you in there yet, because you're visitors at the moment."

The next stop was the third floor. This was the largest unit, with forty beds. The patient load included both medical and surgical patients. Everyone was busy.

"Chapel's down at the end of the hall," Sal said. "You wanna see it?"

I nodded. "Yes, please."

He showed us to a cozy room with beige walls, a double-height ceiling, and wooden chairs with avocado green upholstery. At the inner end was a wooden table for an altar, and two abstract stained-glass windows with a crucifix between them. Being a Catholic, I felt better knowing the chapel was available.

As we walked in, a short, bald man with an olive complexion and dark brown eyes approached us. "Welcome. I'm Father Martin." His smile was like a sudden beam of sunlight illuminating the darkest corners of the room.

Next, Joe took us to a room next to the chapel. His voice was low, almost a whisper. "This is Father Martin's mom. When you're assigned to the third floor, she's gonna be your responsibility."

CHAPTER THREE MOVING FORWARD AFTER SCHOOL

I could only see a head with long gray hair under the covers.

Joe ushered us back out and gently closed the door. "Let's just let her sleep for now."

This time, we took the elevator to the fourth floor and witnessed a quiet unit, much unlike the others. This unit only had twenty beds. At one end a railing opened to the chapel, like a little balcony where a couple of people could sit to participate in the mass.

A gentle voice sounded behind us. "Hi, Joe. How can I help you?"

"These are the new nurses." Joe introduced us to the head nurse, Joanne Lane. She was tall and slender, with brown hair that bounced when she walked. Her eyes were light brown, and she was incredibly soft spoken. I suppose this is why Sister Castille felt the fourth floor was boring. It did not meet her needs for excitement.

The fifth floor housed both medical and surgical patients and was divided into north and south sections. "We're gonna have to blow through here fast." Sal checked his watch. "It's about time for us to get you two down to the office."

As we rode the elevator back down to the first floor, we thanked Sal and Joe for the tour.

"Our pleasure." Joe grinned.

"You bet." Sal gave me his phone number. "Call anytime if you have questions." He winked.

They were both smooth talkers, and when Cassie and I talked about it later, we decided they both had more on their minds than giving a tour. From the kiss placed on our hands, the extensive tour and handing out their phone numbers, it was a bit flirtatious.

In the office, we met with Lucia, who had been a nurse but was now Mrs. Spacha's secretary and the trainer for new nurses.

Lucia took us to a meeting room and gave us a book. "This is our book of policies and procedures. You will need to review it."

We were given two hours to do this, after which we were allowed to go to lunch.

Thanks to Sal's story, Cassie and I hesitated before entering the cafeteria. But we found a table not near the windows and ate a quick lunch. Then we went back upstairs to see Lucia for our next task.

We were asked to demonstrate both intramuscular and subcutaneous injections, as well as starting an IV on a manikin. Next we had to demonstrate CPR on a manikin. We were both nervous with each task, even though we had done these things before. Despite my fluttering nerves, I completed all the tasks effectively, and Cassie did too. By this time, we were exhausted and happy to be finished for the day.

Mrs. Spacha never came out to see us that day.

On day two of orientation, we were expected to complete more reviews of hospital procedures—this time more specific to caring for specific types of situations, such as treating a heart attack, pulmonary embolism (blockage in arteries leading to the lung), umbilical hernia repair, or giving post-operative care to a cholecystectomy (gall bladder removal) patient, and more. We read all day, except during our time for lunch in that wonderful cafeteria.

We spent day three on the unit. Cassie was assigned to five south, and I, to the third floor. Each of us shadowed a nurse, and I was assigned to Edith. She was about my age, slightly overweight, and quick on her feet with short brown hair, blue eyes, and freckles.

A nun called Sister Harriot was working that day as well, and she went with me when I gave my first intramuscular injection on this unit. I had the right medicine, right dose, it was the right time, the right patient, and the right route.

CHAPTER THREE MOVING FORWARD AFTER SCHOOL

I located the site in the right upper gluteal maximus muscle—the right buttocks; this was the easiest site. As I placed my hand in the proper position and cleansed the site with alcohol, Sister Harriot slapped the site. "Now give it," so I did.

Her rationale was that the patient would feel the slap pain, which would offset the injection pain. I'm not so sure about her aseptic technique, though. I am sure one of my nursing instructors would have given her a failing grade for contaminating the injection site.

I felt myself running all day, as opposed to walking. I noticed a blackboard with tasks and room numbers written next to them such as: intake and output, urine testing, IVs, and wound care—to say a few. It all seemed like a blur, but we passed medications, checked IVs, did wound care, passed food trays with the aides, toileted patients, and emptied bedpans and urinals. We had separate clean and dirty holding rooms, and heaven forbid you confuse the two. The clean holding room contained clean linens and supplies while the dirty holding room contained the trash and vessels to empty bedpans and urinals. I noticed a great camaraderie among the staff members, making it a productive working environment.

Taking Charge

After three days of classroom orientation and one day of shadowing the charge nurse, I was assigned to *be* charge nurse. One day shadowing just does not seem to be enough.

I walked into the nurses' station thirty minutes before my shift, ready to hear a report from the day shift. Their report was taped on a cassette recorder—one of those things hospitals no longer use because they've been replaced by higher technology. I went into the adjoining room—the clean holding room—and listened to the report.

That day I was working with one LPN, Sister Roberta, and two aides, Louise and Dina. The unit had two wards with six patients in each, fifteen semiprivate rooms, and of course Father Martin's mother.

Sister Roberta introduced herself. She had been born in Croatia and had a Slavic accent. Her skin was milky white, and she had blue eyes and small features to her face. She wore a full white habit and nursing uniform.

Louise was a tall, black woman, fortyish, with long black hair pulled up in a bun, high cheekbones, and a great complexion. Dina was a white woman, about fifty, with pale skin. Her blue eyes had blood-tinged sclera (the white of the eye). Dina was slender and a few inches shorter than Louise.

Sister Roberta listened to the day shift report with me. The report said six patients were to have either a diagnostic procedure or surgery the next day. The day shift had a unit clerk who made calls and transcribed doctor orders. It was three o'clock in the afternoon, and as the day shift clerk's shift had finished, she had left, even though she had not finished transcribing orders.

The evening shift did not always have a clerk, so the charge nurse—that was me—had to complete those tasks. As I considered the mountain of charts on the desk, I felt a weight, as if a dozen heavy sacks had been laid on my shoulders. I wanted to cry, scream, or run away.

Sister Roberta saw the panic in my eyes. "Let's sit down." She pulled out a chair and sat me down. She explained the process, telling me how to transcribe the orders and get the patients ready for surgery the next day. "Make a list for each patient scheduled for surgery and check off the things you must do—blood work, signed consents, X-Rays, surgical preps, et cetera."

I had done all these things as a student, but this felt different because they were all on my shoulders. And there were so many of them. All at once.

"I will pass medications and do the treatments," Sister Roberta said. "Just notify me if there are any changes in the doctor's orders." She patted my hand. "We will get through this workload together."

CHAPTER THREE MOVING FORWARD AFTER SCHOOL

She was so comforting, and I could not believe I got through all the doctor's orders and completed the lists for all six of the surgical and diagnostic prep patients. I even had time to help with the dinner trays and with getting patients ready for bed, which included repositioning, back rubs, and toileting.

I never went to the cafeteria for dinner, but I gave money to Dina to bring me back a sandwich.

By 10:30 p.m., the only thing left to do was charting on each of my patients for the shift. For example, did they tolerate the new medications, was their appetite good, was their pain relieved, was the surgical wound clean, dry, and intact etc. Sister Roberta did the bulk of it, since she had done the treatments and medications.

As Cassie and I walked out to our cars at the end of our shifts, I learned she had been busy too. On the ride home, I was so tired that I struggled to keep my eyes open.

Chapter Four

REALITY VERSUS SCHOOL

Well, like people say, "Reality sucks."

While the lessons learned in nursing school were the foundation for proficiency in my work, the school workload was nowhere near what I had to do in my job at BCH. To add to that, since I was only making $5.05 per hour, I had to either borrow my dad's car or mooch a ride from Cassie or another friend.

After working for about one month, I had developed somewhat of a routine. I arrived thirty minutes before my evening shift and listened to the day shift report on the tape recorder—or got the information verbally in person if day shift was too busy to tape it—and wrote out tasks for my aides on the blackboard. I did rounds on my patients—thirty to forty of them, depending on the caseload for the day—checking IVs, vital signs, post op dressings, and requests for pain medicine.

Sometimes I worked with Sister Roberta and other times with Jessie, who was also an LPN. She was a black woman who was a little taller than me and was well endowed with a rounded figure. Our second-shift supervisor was Mrs. Thorn, and we were truly blessed having her. Mrs. Thorn had a plump figure and tight curly hair. She wore no makeup—all her beauty shone through her kind and caring face.

CHAPTER FOUR REALITY VERSUS SCHOOL

Doctors Behaving Badly

By now, I was also getting to know the medical residents. One of the memorable residents was Dr. Sojo. His eyes were dark, and with his olive skin tone and a five o'clock shadow, he looked a little too sexy. He introduced himself to me the first time by standing too close for comfort. When he shook my hand, I felt a queasy sensation that worsened after looking into his devilish eyes.

One day while I was standing in the clean holding room listening to the day shift report, I felt him coming up from behind. Thinking he may touch me inappropriately, instinctively, I bent my arms and hit him in the chest with my elbows.

He never tried that again.

But on another occasion, after I assembled supplies for him to perform a blood draw from an artery on a semi-conscious patient, he pulled the curtain around the patient and leaned over to kiss me.

How could he be so bold! I jerked away and stormed out of the room, leaving him to do the procedure on his own. He didn't need the help, but in those days we pampered the doctors, and they expected it.

What made it worse was that, as I walked past the elevator the door opened, and I saw Dr. Kdip embracing another nurse and reaching into her panties. I wanted to throw up.

I ran to Jessie to tell her of my experience. "Can you believe it? Dr. Sojo tried to kiss me over a semiconscious patient! I should report him."

Jessie patted my shoulder. "Honey, no one will do anything about it, so just let it go." She turned back to her chart. "Besides, that man keeps a *sheet* in his car for the nurses who do wanna spend time with him there. So, you know he ain't gonna stop behaving that way."

Ugh! I went into the clean holding room for fifteen minutes, breathing deeply and praying to regain my composure.

45

Two days later, a new male resident started. His name was Dr. Nemi, and he was also very handsome. As he introduced himself, he whispered in my ear, "So, do you burn the candle at both ends." He winked.

I stepped back. "Absolutely not!"

The residents weren't the only feisty ones. One day, as I helped the aides collect urine samples, I approached the patient in bed fourteen and asked for his sample.

He grabbed his urinal and leaped out of bed. Daggers seemed to shoot out of his eyes. Medically, he had a history of paranoid schizophrenia and can only assume he thought I was trying to hurt him.

I ran.

He chased me down the hall.

I found protection behind Jessie.

As the patient approached us, Jessie placed her hands on her hips. "Sucker, you get your ass back in your bed!"

Sheepishly, he walked down the hall to his room and behaved the rest of the night.

Jason

We had quite a variety of patients, ranging in age from twelve to ninety-nine. I loved it when we did have a child, as they were few and far between.

Jason was a little boy I will not forget. He was presented to the hospital with right lower quadrant abdominal pain. He was thirteen years old with black skin, huge dark eyes, a thin body structure, except for a somewhat swollen belly, and an incredibly sad expression.

When I asked his name to confirm I had the right patient, he replied sluggishly. I took his vital signs and examined his belly. When I palpated his belly, he cringed. He still had his clothes on. I suggested he change into a gown. Once he did I could examine the rest of his body, and what I found was devastating.

CHAPTER FOUR REALITY VERSUS SCHOOL

Bruises covered his lower back, and he had a laceration to the back of his head.

My stomach clenched. "What happened here?"

"I fell."

That's what he had also told the emergency room staff. It was the flat way he said it that concerned me. True, I had only been out of nursing school for a few weeks, but my instinct told me something was not right.

I sat next to Jason and, keeping my voice completely calm, asked about the so-called fall.

He looked down. "I can't remember."

Our hospital did not have its own computerized tomography scanner, a machine needed to diagnose appendicitis or an alternate condition. We admitted Jason and, after Dr. Nemi and I finished our assessments, he was quickly transferred to St. Christopher's Hospital for an abdominal CT and then returned.

The CT was negative for an appendicitis, but it showed generalized internal edema (too much fluid was trapped in his body's tissues). Jason's parents were not available. They had dropped him off at the emergency room, told the staff they would return later, and left.

A few minutes after Jason returned from his CT scan, his parents returned. They presented as a well-groomed couple in businesslike attire. The father did all the talking and insisted on a full report of what was done to his son.

I responded, just as businesslike as he, and provided him with all the information I had.

During this conversation, Jason's mother often stared at the floor.

I led them to their son's room. "He's lucky to be alone in a semiprivate room, since our patient count is down today." I pushed open the door and watched anxiously for the son's response to their arrival.

As they entered, Jason caught his mother's eye and grinned. He did not make eye contact with his father.

"Jason, how are you feeling?" Jason's father stepped halfway into the room. "Look at me when I speak to you."

Mom reached for Jason's hand and held it tight.

Quietly, Jason replied, "I'm fine now."

The father glared at me. "Then why is he not discharged?"

"Dr. Linsfield will still need to do an exam on him."

The father grunted. "Well, what are they waiting for? I do not have all day."

"I'll place a call to him and get back with an answer."

"I expect that you should."

I waited until I turned around before I raised my eyebrows and rolled my eyes.

At the nurses' station, I made a call to Dr. Linsfield.

"I'm checking on my post-op patients," he said. "I'll be there in the next two hours."

I was not looking forward to passing this information along to the father, but I stood firmly at the doorway. "Dr. Linsfield is needed with his post-operative patients and will be up here as soon as he can."

The dad was not happy with this, but I did not stay in the room to wait for another remark.

When Dr. Linsfield arrived at my unit, I pulled him aside to let him know my concerns that this may be a case of child abuse. He agreed he would address the bruises.

I walked with Dr. Linsfield to the room. He introduced himself kindly but firmly to the parents first. "Oh, you must be Jason. I hear you have a bit of a bellyache."

Jason smiled. "It did hurt, but it's gone now."

Dr. Linsfield made small talk with him and then examined his belly. "Turn over, please." He studied Jason's back a moment. "Mom, Dad, look at this please." He pointed to the bruises and stepped back so they could see.

CHAPTER FOUR REALITY VERSUS SCHOOL

"He fell," the father snapped.

Dr. Linsfield and I both noticed that a tear leaked from one of the mother's eyes.

"Jason, how did you fall?" Dr. Linsfield asked.

"I fell down the stairs. Cut my head too."

"I see." Dr. Linsfield looked at the laceration, then turned to the parents. "I will check his labs and CT scan and advise you of my recommendations."

"I don't think so," the father boomed.

"I do." Dr. Linsfield walked out.

Anger flashed in the father's eyes. "We'll be back in the morning." They left.

I received orders to clean the laceration on Jason's head and draw more labs. While I did these things, I chatted and joked with him, making him smile. Dr. Linsfield ordered a psychologist to talk to Jason, and Dr. Pringle was called.

Following his evaluation of Jason, Dr. Pringle met with Dr. Linsfield and me at the nurses' station. He sighed. "Jason does not show sufficient evidence of being an abused child—"

"How is that possible?" I squealed.

Dr. Linsfield patted my shoulder.

Dr. Pringle nodded as if he understood what I meant. "But it does appear that he lacks a tender, loving relationship with his father. It may even be somewhat neglectful."

That seemed to me a gross understatement, but what could I do? Nothing but shake with rage.

The next morning when Jason' parents arrived, Dr. Linsfield made it a point to be there, so he could go over the test results with them. He told them all was stable, and Jason could go home.

I talked more with Dr. Pringle about this later.

"Your instincts are a great tool," he said, "and you had every right to be concerned. But there was not enough evidence to file a report. But all of our findings are in his record now, so if Jason should come in again with a similar type of injury, a report to child protective services may have more weight."

Prepping Poop Patients

Three common diagnoses on our unit were acute cholecystitis (inflamed gall bladder), acute pancreatitis (inflammation of the pancreas) and acute diverticulitis (inflammation on the inside wall of the intestines). I gave more suppositories, enemas, and cleansing agents than I care to admit to so physicians could fully examine patients' innards.

The common tests were either an upper or lower gastrointestinal (GI) series; the former was done with a barium swallow and the latter with a barium enema completed in the radiology department. Barium is a mineral that shows up on Xrays, so when it's introduced into the body, it allows the digestive tract to be examined.

The upper GI series had little prep involving a liquid diet and "NPO after midnight." Like a lot of medical jargon, this comes from Latin: *nil per os* means *nothing by mouth*, so in other words it indicates that the patient can have nothing to eat or drink.

But oh, the lower GI series was the deluxe test. At times, we had as many as eight steps for barium enemas. We would start with the bottle of magnesium citrate, a laxative, then tablets that contained a different laxative, and finally a suppository by 8 p.m. If the patient had no results by 10 p.m., we had to give a tap water enema until the results were clear. These were the times, I wished we had showers for the nurses because the scent of poop was upon us.

Coming into second shift the next day, we were faced with ten patients who had undergone barium swallows or enemas earlier in the day. All that wonderful white barium had to come out sometime. We spent the entire shift either running patients to the bathroom or putting them on bedpans. Sister Roberta, Louise, and I felt like we were filming a comedy scene for *I Love Lucy* as we transferred these patients back and forth from bed to bathroom. We reeked of poop.

Informed Consent

The next day, we were prepping some of these patients for surgery. This was becoming more of a routine for me since my tutoring from Sister Roberta.

As usual, many of the surgical consent forms were not completed during the day shift, leaving me to sit with these patients, reviewing the procedures with them, and obtaining their written consents.

I made sure the pre-op medications were received from the pharmacy, checked that all the labs were done, as well as chest Xrays and electrocardiograms, with results in the chart. Medical clearances were completed as needed.

Time was of the essence in completing all preoperative tasks, but at times we would have to spend additional time on issues such as women refusing to remove jewelry or nail polish. Fortunately, I learned we could tape around rings for those who either refused to take off their rings or if a ring was physically impossible to remove. Regarding the women who refused to have their nail polish removed, we had to explain that since they were unable to communicate while under anesthesia, the surgical team would monitor blood flow in their fingertips to ensure it was all right.

Even though we had physical and occupational therapists working with some of the patients, the nurse was responsible to make sure bedbound patients received range of motion exercises and frequent repositioning and that those who were ambulatory (able to walk) took an occasional stroll to prevent contractures (shortening of muscles) or bedsores and to reduce the risk of pneumonia.

The patient in bed six was a twenty-five-year-old woman who, I was told by the day shift staff, was a lady of the evening. She was emaciated, pale, and unkempt. Day shift's report indicated that a cab had dropped her off after

Nursing, Yes I Do!

she had been beaten by an unknown man. She had bruises all over her body, and the laceration to her forehead was so deep that the emergency room physician had placed a Penrose drain. This drain is a soft, flexible rubber tube used to prevent the buildup of fluid in an injury or surgical site, allowing fluid to drain outside the skin to a piece of gauze.

This patient needed a CT scan of her head to check for a potential brain injury. Because that would be done at another hospital, she would need to sign a consent form permitting the transfer, as well as the scan. I prepared the forms and explained to her that she would have a special Xray with a machine that we did not have in our hospital. She narrowed her eyes and cocked her head to the side.

I continued by saying, "This machine will take pictures of your brain to tell us if there was any injury."

"Can I bring my panties?"

"Yes, you can, but do you understand what I am saying?"

She again looked at me in confusion.

At this point I began to use my hands in my description, pointing to my head from both sides. "The CT scan machine is large and has many little cameras that will take pictures of your brain. It won't hurt, and you'll return back here after the test."

She again looked at me with her forehead wrinkled. "Can I bring my panties?"

I did not realize that Mrs. Thorn had been standing behind me the whole time until she put her hand on my shoulder and said gently, "Just give her the consent and pen and instruct her to sign it."

I did as she asked. Mission accomplished.

Adventuresome Patients

Nothing was like the wards. We had two of them, one with women and one with men. You could enter one to change an IV and not leave

CHAPTER FOUR REALITY VERSUS SCHOOL

for a half hour because of multiple questions, requests for pain shots, complaints about roommates, and taking time to redirect patients with dementia.

My favorite episode in the ward was when Mr. Pope in Bed C went to the extreme in trying to escape from his posey restraint jacket. This is a sleeveless garment with long wide ties at shoulders and waist, allowing you to tie a patient to a chair to prevent him or her from falling or wandering.

This little emaciated man was very confused and continually tried to escape from his room. Because he needed assistance to walk to prevent him from falling, we had to apply this restraint when he was in his chair or bed. I know it sounds harsh to tie someone up, but we visited him frequently to make sure he knew we did not forget him and to ensure he was not hurting himself with the restraints. We put him in a high-back geriatric chair, which is like a recliner on wheels. Often we saw him shimmy the chair across the floor by rocking it. He was a strong little guy.

One day between our checks, we heard him yelling, which was not unusual. But this time he sounded different. Jessie went to the ward, and there he was in his chair, which had tipped over. The top of the chair back was on the floor and the bottom of the chair faced the ceiling. Mr. Pope was hanging upside down, still tied in his posey, his head just inches from the floor. He apparently shimmied too much and toppled the chair.

We rushed to his side and held in our laughter until we got him upright. He just kept screaming, and we told him to stop so we could assess him.

No injuries, thank heaven.

Poseys are rarely used anymore, because if a patient is not monitored regularly in a posey, the person can strangle himself or herself.

Nursing, Yes I Do!

One Sunday in the last quarter of my shift, I thought all was calm.

Then Louise ran into the nurses' station yelling, "The patient from room fourteen is headed down the street!"

I exclaimed, "What?"

She repeated it, and I ran to the stairwell and looked out the window. Sure enough, there she was walking down the street. I ran outside as quickly as I could to reach her. I caught up to her and then, trying to catch my breath, I pleaded with her to come back with me.

"No," she snapped, "I need to go back to Tennessee to see my family."

"We can call them from the nurses' station."

No luck. I was not about to physically pull her back, so I ran back to the nurses' station.

In the interim, Jessie had called security. They in turn called the police to pick her up.

Within thirty minutes, she had been evaluated by Dr. Kdip and was back in her bed with no recollection of what she had done.

As I was getting her settled for the night, I bent down to raise the head of the bed with that lovely manual crank.

Dr. Kdip goosed me.

I whipped around. "Do not ever do that again."

He just laughed and walked out of the room.

I had some good times with the girls on the third floor. We talked about food, parties, men, and our bodies. "My breasts are so small," I moaned.

Jessie, in her usual blunt manner, proclaimed, "Honey, you gotta have your man suck on those boobs."

My jaw dropped. I think I turned various shades of red. Then I laughed with the rest of the girls in the nurses' station.

CHAPTER FOUR REALITY VERSUS SCHOOL

During one spell, we were regularly receiving the supper trays around 6 p.m.—thirty minutes past the time we should have gotten them.

One day, while discussing this problem with my all-black female aide group, I blurted, "I cannot believe our floor is always so late. It is as if we are on the blacklist."

I remember casually turning around and going back to work, but later I feared I might have said something wrong. I loved those girls, and we worked and communicated together well. It turns out that, etymologically, the word *blacklist* isn't related to Black people, but at the time I worried I had misspoken.

After we passed out the trays, I thought I should ask whether or not I had offended them. They often sat in the dirty holding room for a cigarette break while the patients were eating, which was fine, as long as no call bells chimed.

I walked into the dirty holding room. Louise was sitting there with a couple of the other girls.

"About what I said earlier." I kneaded my hands. "I'm sorry . . . I hope I didn't offend anyone when I said *blacklist*."

Louise blew out a stream of smoke and shrugged. "We never heard that term before."

"Oh. As I understand it, it means certain people are negatively targeted."

They laughed, and I did too, and we went on with our work.

State Boards

I had something else to be concerned about now. It was time to take the state nursing board exams. I had been studying a couple of hours most mornings before my shift and two to four hours on my days off. The exams were given twice per year over a two-day period. There were five sections: Medical, Surgical, OB/GYN, Pediatrics, and Psychiatry.

Cassie, Rhonda, Missy, Penny, Corrine, and I were scheduled to take the exams in Niagara Falls and had booked hotel rooms. I was rooming with Corrine.

Toward the end of October, we arrived in the late afternoon the day before the exam. The six of us decided to drive together in Penny's car. She had a station wagon that fit us all comfortably. The sky was still light out, and the trees glowed with autumnal colors. We laughed almost all the way through the car ride, except it was that nervous laughter. Obviously, we were all a bit uptight.

At the hotel, we noticed many girls and boys we believed were there for the testing, too. After dinner, we took our showers, put on our jammies, and headed to Cassie and Missy's room to go over a few things before the exam.

The topic we chose was infant development, with emphasis on the reflexes. We laid on Cassie's bed mimicking these. Silly as it sounds, this helped us remember them.

One is the tonic neck reflex, which is when a baby turns the head to one side, and the arm on that side extends out while the other arm pulls in. It looks kind of like a little cupid about to shoot an arrow from a bow. Another is the Moro reflex, which happens when a baby's head position shifts suddenly. The child will flail the arms out, then pull them back in again.

We laughed at each other because of how silly we looked imitating infants with their arms bent this way and that way so we could demonstrate the reflexes correctly. After only thirty minutes, we decided if we didn't know these things by now, we would be out of luck. We decided to hit the sack.

Corrine and I said only a few words to each other before we drifted off the sleep.

Beeeeep . . .

CHAPTER FOUR REALITY VERSUS SCHOOL

Corrine and I both sat up like a bolt of lightning hit us. It was 6 a.m. and time to get ready for our first day of exams. We were all dressed and downstairs in fifteen minutes for our continental breakfast and coffee. That morning was quite different from the night before, as we barely spoke.

A shuttle took us to the convention center, where the exams were being given. The ride only took five minutes, but it seemed like an hour.

Once we got inside, about 200 other nursing graduates joined us. I picked up my identification badge and two pencils and headed to my seat. Knowing we were not allowed to bring in purses, I had left mine in my room. Lockers were available for people who had brought theirs.

The room looked cold and unwelcoming, with high steel-beamed ceilings and thin gray carpeting. We were assigned seats in alphabetical order. The desks were like you would see in school—hard and uncomfortable. Middle-aged proctors stood at the front of every row with booklets in their hands.

After about five minutes, a voice cracked over the intercom. "Applicants, please be quiet."

The two days of exams dragged, and I was elated when they were over. I really was not sure how I did. I just hoped I passed.

Comfort Zone

After only a couple of months at BCH, I received a raise, bringing me up to $5.55 per hour. This gave me a warm feeling of acceptance.

Occasionally, I filled in on the fourth floor—the quiet one. I worked with one aide, and believe me, that was all I needed to care for the ten patients. At times, the supervisor took the aide to use on another floor. That was fine because I could handle it myself.

Sister Castille was part-time supervisor on the days Mrs. Thorn was off. I enjoyed working with both. Sister Castille made me laugh sometimes when she complained of a slow-moving shift. I would think, *Why would a nun be wishing for more action?*

I would walk down the hall making my rounds and often sat on the balcony and overlooked the chapel. Sometimes, Father Martin came and sat with me, and we would chat for an hour or so. That's how quiet it was.

One day, when I was assigned to the fourth floor, the day nurse gave me her report and then, when she got to the end, she grew quiet. "And, uh, lastly, Sal is here."

"What? Sal the ambulance attendant?"

"Yeah. He . . . was the driver on a run, and he . . . struck a small child that ran out into the street."

"Oh, no," I whispered.

"The child was severely injured but is expected to make it."

"Well, that's something. And Sal?"

She took a deep breath, as if steeling herself. "Sal had a nervous breakdown. That's why he was admitted to our unit."

Denise was a part-time nurse frequently assigned to the fourth floor but not scheduled for the next couple of days. Since she had been a close friend of Sal, she came in on her day off to sit with him. She spent most of the shift in his room with the door closed, coming out only to retrieve his medications and food trays.

Sal was discharged after a couple of days but didn't return to work for several weeks. I did learn that the injured child's condition stabilized, and he was discharged from the hospital after a few days, but I never heard the specifics of his injuries.

Disappointment

In December, that long-awaited response from the State Board of Education came in the mail. I held my breath and opened the envelope ever so slowly.

CHAPTER FOUR REALITY VERSUS SCHOOL

As I read the results, a burning sensation developed in my chest, followed by a shiver down my spine.

I had passed the medical, surgical, and OB/GYN sections. I had failed the pediatrics and psychiatry sections. I would have to repeat them in March. Until then, I was still a Graduate Nurse.

I called Cassie. "How did you do?"

"I passed all five sections!"

"Good for you!" I meant it. "Congratulations!"

Of the six who had driven to Niagara in Penny's station wagon, I was the only one who did not pass all five sections.

I felt totally deflated.

Chapter 5

WEDDING PREPARATIONS

I found solace in my mother and my fiancé, Ethan. And I dealt with the blow of not passing all my boards by shifting gears to my wedding, which was approaching in the next few months. I still had much to do and did not want to ruin my wedding day by feeling depressed.

The next day, I gave my results to my supervisor Mrs. Thorn. She was so understanding. "You will pass next time," she reassured.

I prayed she was right. It was time for a review, and despite my exam results, I was still given a raise for the good work I did. I was now up to $6.05 an hour.

Christmas was the following week, and I would work my usual evening shift on Christmas Eve and New Year's Day. Full-timers had to work two out of the four holidays, and I lucked out. A lot of food was flowing into the units from co-workers, and we found ourselves unit-hopping, sharing the food and festivities.

I heard through the grapevine that a new nurse was being hired, and I hoped I would be transferred to five north. This unit had only thirty patients, although five south had sixteen. Either unit would have been an improvement from the forty-bed third floor.

First Transfer

My wish came true, and I was transferred up to five north. I missed working with Sister Roberta and Jessie, but I would still see them, either

CHAPTER 5 WEDDING PREPARATIONS

on break or passing. On five north, I worked with either Sandy or Sister Harriot. Sandy was a tall, blonde, slender girl who loved to add salt to her already salted potato chips. How she stayed so thin, I will never know. I enjoyed working with her because she was kind, intelligent, easy to talk to, and a hard worker. Sandy and I took turns as charge nurse while the others passed medications and did treatments.

Sister Harriot was originally from a small country in Eastern Europe and had come to the United States to escape religious persecution. She never spoke of any details, but her coarse exterior let us know she was hurting inside. She stood only five feet tall, with a round body, and she wore the full white habit. When she arrived for her shift, she would listen to the report and then say each time, as if I would not remember, "You take charge; I do meds and go to chapel."

I would always respond, "Yes, Sister."

The aides often floated from floor to floor, so at times I saw Louise or Joanne or worked with one of the other third-floor aides.

We had a little more down time on five north than on the third floor, and it was welcomed because when we worked, we worked hard.

I spent a good amount of time giving pain shots on this floor. I recall that one of my patients who had been discharged after a cholecystectomy (gall bladder removal) called our unit asking me to bring a pain shot to his house. Seriously!

Now, on the other hand, one individual really needed the pain shot, and I had to practically demand it from the doctor. The patient in room five by the door was admitted with a crushed right foot. He had been running over a set of train tracks when he tripped and fell. His right foot had become caught in between the railroad ties. After several minutes he was able to loosen his foot, seconds before a train approached. But his foot had crushing injuries from the pressure he exerted while trying to release

Nursing, Yes I Do!

it from the railroad ties. To his benefit, he had consumed enough whiskey before the incident to lessen the pain.

I completed my assessment and, upon looking at the foot, I held my gasp until after I returned to the nurses' station. All of the toes were almost flattened, and bruised to the extent that they were barely recognizable. He would obviously need an amputation.

He had tears in his eyes from the pain, and he screamed in agony.

Dr. Saki, one of our surgical residents, wrote the admission orders and only prescribed Tylenol with codeine for the pain. This obviously would not touch his pain.

I called Dr. Saki, asking for a stronger pain medication.

He asked, "Well how much pain is he in?"

"Hold on." I carried the phone out into the hall. "Here. Listen."

The man's screams could well be heard on the phone.

"I'm sorry," Dr. Saki said. "Because I was called away for an incoming motor vehicle accident involving three victims, I was unable to complete a full assessment on this man when he presented to the emergency room. Give him Dilaudid, one to two milligrams intramuscularly, beginning now. I'll be up to re-evaluate him later this evening."

I thanked Dr. Saki on behalf of the patient—and everyone else on the floor, for that matter. The patient in turn thanked me over and over after I gave him the pain shot. Within ten minutes, he was asleep.

Sandy was getting floated off of five north more often, so at times I would work with Maryanne. Like Sandy, Maryanne was tall. How I wished even two inches could be added to my mere five-foot stature. At any rate, Maryanne had short, curly, dark brown hair, unusually pale skin, and though she was more serious than Sandy, she was still easy to communicate with.

CHAPTER 5 WEDDING PREPARATIONS

"You won't believe what happened yesterday," Maryanne said one day. I had been off the day before. "Oh? What?"

"I misplaced a page off the IV board."

"That doesn't sound too bad." I mean, it wasn't good, but... you see, every patient with an intravenous (IV) line had a written page for each IV fluid that was being given. We kept these lists on a clipboard and used it to check each IV and monitor the flow and mark the amount infused each shift. So, it was important. But one page misplaced for a short time shouldn't have been a big deal.

"You have no idea. Sister Harriot took the board from me and hit me over the head with it. "You stupid, stupid girl," she said. My sides hurt from holding my laughter in.

The next day, I found Sister Harriot standing on a chair in the nurses' station. "A mouse! I saw a mouse!" She clutched the skirts of her habit.

It was my turn to hold in laughter while I searched for—but did not find—a mouse. I took Sister's hand to help her down from the chair.

On occasion, I was floated to five south. What a cake job. There were only eight semiprivate rooms, and the patients were primarily medical problems rather than surgical.

On one such occasion, I had a new admission coming in at 4 p.m.—a forty-year-old male being admitted with acute pancreatitis.

"Hi, I'm Aubrey. I'll be looking after you today." I attempted to begin my assessment, but he stopped me.

"I have to make a call. You can come back later."

When I returned to his room, I took his vital signs. "Do you have any symptoms I should know about?"

"I have to make another call."

"All right." Since he had arrived so close to dinner, he would not be able to order a specific dinner from the kitchen. So, I snuck in a quick question.

"Shall I order you a sandwich, or will a dinner tray of turkey, mashed potatoes, and beans be acceptable?"

"Just give me the dinner tray."

I left him to make his call. Later I brought his tray in.

"What the f--- is this? I will not eat this crap."

Three times, I opened my mouth and tried to say I would call the kitchen and see what else they had, but each time, he cut me off and yelled at me.

"Let me know when you are ready to discuss this." I spun around, and as I left the room, his tray followed me out the door, just missing my head.

Before I could get to my phone to call for security, two police officers were already barreling down the hall. Working the evening shift, we were blessed with city police on site, based on the frequent hostilities that occurred.

I pointed to the room, and when they entered, I heard a scuffle.

The officers exited the room with that patient in handcuffs, squirming, and yelling.

Two hours later, the two police officers returned. "Would you be willing to testify about this incident if necessary? Because the patient claimed security beat him up."

"Of course, I will."

Re-Take of the State Boards

For three months, I had studied like a maniac to pass the remaining two sections of the state boards. I really felt confident this time, but the whole idea of being in that huge room with that huge book of questions put my stomach in knots. Each section had 150 questions.

I tossed the problem around for a bit and finally decided to ask my doctor for a prescription for Valium for a couple of days.

Exam day arrived, and I was back in Niagara Falls—alone this time. Since the tests were both on the same day, I could take them and go home, instead of staying overnight in a hotel.

CHAPTER 5 WEDDING PREPARATIONS

As I approached the convention center, I felt a lump in my throat but quickly talked myself out of being upset. I had taken the Valium the prior day and one that morning. It was a low dose and did not make me drowsy.

I found an empty desk and noticed a classmate of mine. We exchanged winks and a whispered "good luck."

The proctor passed out the packets. I watched as the clock finally reached 9 a.m. A bell rang, jangling my nerves. I tore open the packet and began.

Up first: pediatrics. I took my time reading the questions but did not read anything over and over. I finished about fifteen minutes before the time was up.

With an hour to go before the psychiatric section exam, I went to get some lunch.

I noticed that classmate again, and we walked to the café and had lunch together.

""I had to come back from North Carolina to re-take the pediatric and psychiatric sections," she said.

"North Carolina!" My day trip hardly seemed an inconvenience compared to that.

My Stagette

My wedding was approaching, and the staff wanted to take me out for drinks. I was ready. Our police officers arranged it—a coed stagette.

It was a cool Friday evening in early April 1978, and we headed to a corner bar two blocks away. Fifteen people from the hospital joined me to celebrate.

I lost myself in conversation with friends, had two cocktails and a cigarette, and then decided to ask for something heavy duty. I captured the bartender's attention. "Make me a godfather"—a mix of scotch and amaretto.

Nursing, Yes I Do!

"No." The bartender grinned. "You should have a honeymoon cocktail." He grabbed one bottle after another, dashing a variety of unknown liquors into a cocktail shaker, smirking as he shook his mixture with extra panache. He slid a martini glass across the polished bar top and, with a flourish, proceeded to pour absolutely nothing into it.

I laughed.

"You really do not want to get drunk, do you?" He was acting as my guardian angel so that I did not make a fool of myself.

The evening was over before I knew it.

The Burn Unit

I had been curious about the burn unit—more commonly called the BTC—ever since Sal and Joe had shown it to me on my initial tour.

One day, I was asked to cover dinner hour for the burn unit girls because one of them was celebrating a birthday, and they all wanted to go together.

At the door, I pressed the buzzer. "This is Aubrey."

The door clicked, and I pushed it open. This was my first real involvement with the nurses in this unit. The BTC had its own supervisor, Fran Dolski. Today was not the day to meet her though. The routine evening nurses were Jackie and Janet.

Jackie, a brunette with a fair complexion, was thin and a little taller than me. She gave me a gown to wear over my uniform. As I put it on, she laid out a mask, cap, and gloves. "You'll only need to use these if there's an emergency."

Janet was the same height, with dirty blond hair. She struck me as somewhat mysterious. "Just stay in the nurses' station. If any of the patients call on the intercom asking for more pain medication, tell them they are on schedule to receive it soon."

"But I can—"

CHAPTER 5 WEDDING PREPARATIONS

"Nope." Janet shook her head. "All of these patients have extreme pain, and they are all on a strict schedule."

I nodded. "Okay, I get it." The heaviest-duty pain shots have to be administered carefully, or they can do more harm than good.

Jackie handed me a card. "Just in case there is an emergency, here are our pager numbers."

They left, and my heart sank into my stomach. I prayed no one would call and nothing horrible would happen while I sat there.

One patient's room was directly across from the nurses' station in immediate view. I peered in and saw a woman covered in gauze from her neck down to her toes. Her arms were strung up from IV poles with more gauze, one on each side, to elevate the wounds.

Within a few minutes, she began to swing her arms around as if she were taking flight and began to shriek like a chicken. "Bock, bock, bock, bock."

My eyes widened and this time, my stomach felt like it jumped into my throat. *She is not hurting herself . . . her arms are still tied . . . the gauze is still intact.*

This lasted for about ten minutes. I guess she got tired and stopped.

I walked around the nurses' station and read the signs posted, the brochures, and briefly a couple of charts specific to how the patients were burned. Reading about the severity of their injuries and the meticulous nature of their treatments caused my heart to ache for them.

Before I knew it, Jackie and Janet returned. I told them about the chicken lady.

They just laughed. Jackie said, "She does that all the time."

As I left the BTC, I thought about the extreme needs of these patients, and others like them. My heart bloomed with a yearning for critical care nursing.

Wedding and Honeymoon

Well, that special day finally arrived. I woke up with a soaring feeling of elation and headed downstairs to the kitchen. I felt like I was floating on air and gave my parents a loving hug.

The time before the ceremony flew by, with the myriad of preparation activities: hair and nail appointments, photographs with my parents and my bridal attendants, and the limousine ride to the church.

The ceremony and the reception went without a hitch, and we headed to our long-awaited honeymoon in Hawaii. Truly an amazing place and better than I anticipated.

After a glorious week, it was time to get back to reality and to work.

The Move

After one year, I wanted to get off the evening shift. And now that I was married, I really wanted to be on the same shift as my husband. Mrs. Thorn was extremely impressed with my work and immediately put my request through.

In addition to this, the hospital would be moving to a new building just beyond the parking lot. A very generous family had given a multimillion-dollar donation for a new hospital.

All the staff had to help pack supplies. We used garbage totes for many of the supplies, as they were large and easy to transport across the parking lot. The National Guard came in to help transport the critical patients, and the others were transported by van or by wheelchair. Some even walked over, with our assistance. It was quite a sight.

Morning meds were passed at the old place and afternoon meds at the new place. There was quite a bit of confusion the first twenty-four hours, but no mistakes were made.

CHAPTER 5 WEDDING PREPARATIONS

My new unit was the fifth floor. No more split floors of north and south. The main floor was billing, clinics, emergency room, and a small prayer room for Father Martin. I felt sad for him because they had promised him a chapel, even though it would be smaller than the old one. But he got a meager ten-by-ten-foot room.

Surgery and the BTC were on the second floor. The ICU (Intensive Care Unit) and administration offices were on the third floor. The fourth floor was for patients scheduled for surgery, and the fifth floor was for patients who needed monitoring and non-surgical care.

There was an opening for a registered nurse in the intensive care unit. I really enjoyed working as a nurse and was eager to learn more, so I jumped at the chance to work there. I discussed it with Ms. Thorn. The timing was perfect, as I had just received news that I had passed the state boards and was officially a registered nurse (RN). I could not stop looking at my license. With this, I received another raise, so I was up to $6.55 per hour.

The following Saturday I was off, and Ethan and I were invited to a barbecue at Cassie's boyfriend Andrew's house—or should I say his parents' house. It was a beautiful day, and the guests included some from the hospital, some of his family and our college buddies, Penny, Rhonda, Corrine, and Missy. We had a great time.

During this party Cassie and Andrew announced their engagement. I was so happy for them! It was a day for celebration.

Then I learned that Andrew was entering medical school in about a year, which would take him and Cassie to San Francisco. I would really miss her.

Intensive Care Unit

Great news! Ms. Thorn called me to tell me I was granted the position to work in the ICU. "You're obviously doing a good job," she said, "and management respects you."

Nursing, Yes I Do!

On my first day in ICU, I was introduced to the staff and shadowed Barbara. She had light skin and stood about half a foot taller than me. She had tightly cut,, short blond hair, a slightly plump figure, and spoke with a brassy tone. Without much preliminary conversation, she called me into room seven to help her dress a wound.

Upon entering the room, I saw a middle-aged black female, barely responsive, on oxygen, with a large dressing to her right inner thigh.

Barbara took her right leg and lifted it high. "Dress this wound."

I looked at her, then at the patient, who was moaning and shifting, in obvious discomfort. "What's the patient's name?" I asked.

"It's Mrs. J., now hurry up."

"Hi, Mrs. J. I'm Aubrey. I'll take care of this for you." I washed my hands, then gathered sponge pads, tape, saline, and the ointment Barbara instructed me to use.

While I removed the old dressing, I spoke to Mrs. J., telling her what I was doing. I stifled my gasp as I unveiled the wound. I could have fit my entire hand into it.

After I completed the task, I smiled at Mrs. J., and she smiled back.

"I'll check on you soon," I said.

The head nurse's name was Judy. All of her features were tiny, but she had a manly, deep voice. Her initial comment to me was, "You better get used to dealing with stabbings, shootings, junkies, and drug dealers in here."

Adele was a full-time aide and probably the most beautiful lady working at the hospital. Her skin was the color of cream, her loosely curled blond hair fell about mid-neck length, and her smile could melt an ice cube. I enjoyed working with her tremendously.

Because these patients needed a higher level of care, we did what we call primary nursing, as opposed to team nursing on the floor. Each nurse would be assigned two to four patients and did everything for them:

CHAPTER 5 WEDDING PREPARATIONS

personal care, medications, IVs, and treatments, with help from the aide. Their ICU could house only eight patients.

Days passed, and before I knew it, I could take the charge nurse position, if Judy and Barbara were off, and work with the float staff.

My role as charge nurse included getting the report from the night charge nurse. My support staff of nurses and aides was also present for the report. At times we completed the report while making rounds to a particular patient's room, checking his or her IVs, ventilator settings, surgical sites, and drainage tubes as needed.

I would in turn assign patients to my nursing staff. We were only provided one aide, and my nurses would give the aide tasks to do, which generally involved bathing, dressing, emptying drainage bags, passing food trays, and feeding those who were allowed to eat.

If I did not make rounds with the night shift charge nurse, I did so on my own, visiting each patient to reassure myself they were stable.

We needed another full-time nurse in the ICU, so on the days when I was in charge, I worked with two nurses who floated from the medical or surgical floors.

One day as I was making rounds, I entered the room of a new admission: a male patient brought in a couple of hours earlier with a gunshot wound to the chest.

An inadequate 4-inch-by-4-inch sponge dressing was partially taped over the wound, but it blew in and out on the breeze caused by the patient's breathing.

I leaned back into the hall. "I need a doctor in here and a chest tube tray!"

One of the house physicians sprinted in, and an aide brought the tray. Working quickly, we put in a chest tube to drain fluid from the wound and sealed the chest with a suitably sized dressing. It's not an exaggeration to say this treatment saved the man's life.

Nursing, Yes I Do!

The unit was pretty secure, and no one would expect a patient to go missing, but in bed five was a tall male patient, who decided he wanted to leave. He opened the stairwell door and headed down the steps. Fortunately, I saw him and followed.

Regrettably, once those stairwell doors closed, someone in the hall outside had to let you back in. Otherwise, the only way out was to go all the way down to the first floor and exit there.

I kept talking to him all the way down, pleading with him to stop. I stayed close, hoping to break his fall, if it should happen.

His only response was, "I would rather die at home."

Once we reached the first floor, I opened the door and waved to a nearby office worker. "Call security."

She did, and together the guard and I got him into a wheelchair and took him back upstairs.

I gave him his sedative and called the house staff physician to check him out as well. Fortunately, he was okay.

When we had down time, I loved chatting with Adele. She was an obviously great cook, based on the recipes she would tell me about. I give credit to her on instructing me how to make turkey gravy, although at times it did not turn out quite right.

After a couple of months, a new nurse was hired. Janice was an extremely attractive, fair-complexioned, tall, slender girl with blonde hair and blue eyes. She graduated from Christolette College with me, but I did not really know her.

I did know she was a good friend with Rosanne. Janice told me that after graduation, she and Rosanne had gone down to Florida, and both

CHAPTER 5 WEDDING PREPARATIONS

had been hired at the same hospital. Rosanne had kept up her drug addiction. One day the head nurse approached Rosanne, who was obviously high, and pulled her off the floor. Janice said she had never heard anything else from Rosanne after that.

It was a joy working with Janice, and we became close. Our work was done without a hitch, and I noticed a softening of both Judy and Barbara. Janice and I went out for a drink a few times after work to relieve our stress. But just as quickly as she appeared, she was gone. She worked with us for two months, and then we never heard from her again.

When Janice left, Maryanne came down to ICU, and we picked up our relationship from when we worked together before. I was getting skeptical about getting close to anyone, so I kept this relationship purely work related. Cassie was still my buddy, and we would get together sometimes after work for a cocktail, but I had to steel myself for the time she would move to San Francisco. Cassie had been filling in as part-time supervisor around her shifts in the emergency room. I truly felt happy for her.

No matter how many times I responded to a code, it never got easier on the mind.

On an otherwise quiet Sunday morning, the cardiac monitor alarm in room three went off. Judy, Barbara, and I ran into the room to find the patient on the floor leaning against the bed. The monitor read zero.

We gently laid him flat on the floor. We found no pulse or respiration. Barbara pulled the code button to summon the team. Judy placed a backboard under his chest for support. We began cardiopulmonary resuscitation (CPR), with me applying chest compressions while Barbara used an ambu bag (a mask with an air bag attached) to pump air into the patient's lungs.

Nursing, Yes I Do!

The team arrived, with Father Martin close behind. He would usually respond by giving blessings and last rites if needed. This time, Father Martin got in the way a bit.

Judy was upset, so she stepped on his hand. "Sorry, Father, but please move."

We worked on this thirty-eight-year-old heart attack victim for forty-five minutes with no success.

Dr. Sojo called it to stop and pronounced the patient dead at 10:48 a.m.

We rolled a sheet under him, lifted him up to the bed and cleaned him up just in time for the arrival of his wife and parents.

I met them in the hall and broke the news. "I'm so sorry for your loss." Then I led them into the room. The task of giving more specifics about his condition had fallen to me, but no matter what you say, it is always received in disbelief. "The doctor is at the desk, and he'll be in shortly to see you and answer more of your questions."

I stepped out, closing the door to give them more privacy. Down the hall, I reminded Dr. Sojo that the family was waiting for him. I could hear their weeping from our desk.

Shortly thereafter, he walked down to the room and shut the door behind him.

Chapter 6

WORKING THE BURN UNIT

After six months I felt a strong desire to work in the burn unit. I was still working day shift, and a position was open in the unit. Again, I spoke with Mrs. Thorn, who was now day shift supervisor, and she was happy to oblige.

My first burn unit shift was on a Friday, and the unit had just admitted two new patients.

Laura was still the head nurse, and the supervisor was still Fran Dolski. Laura's umber complexion was flawless, and she carried herself like a runway model. Her smile could light up the room. Fran looked more businesslike, with her three-piece suits and wearing just enough make-up to highlight her high cheekbones and huge green eyes.

Day shift nurses included Vanessa and Stella. Vanessa could have passed as Lucy Arnaz in her looks and personality. Stella was of Polish descent, and while she spoke English, she had a distinct accent. Marge was our housekeeper and also functioned as an aide. Marge was large, rugged, and carried a musty odor. We disregarded the odor because she worked so hard. Occasionally, a secretary floated to our unit, or the charge nurse carried these duties.

Jackie and Janet were the evening nurses. They were as opposite in looks and personality as night and day, but that did not interfere with their work. Jackie was as prim and proper as an English duchess, while Janet presented herself as a call girl.

Nelson and Pam were the night nurses. Nelson stood over six feet and had striking dark wavy hair and dark eyes. He carried an extra talent of singing country and western songs with a band and had occasional gigs before his night shift.

Pam was a new graduate awaiting the results of her boards. She had moved there from Florida with her fiancé because of his job transfer. She had the most amazing golden blonde curly hair, which blended in with her light complexion and small stature.

The unit had three phase one beds and ten phase two beds. Laura took me on a tour of the unit. She first showed me the equipment, including the saline warmer. All burn patients had to have their wounds initially cleansed with saline, which needed to be warm. Gauze of all shapes and sizes was stored in the clean holding room.

The refrigerator had the homograft, and the freezer had the xenograft tissue. Heaven forbid you should mix them up. Xenograft tissue, also called heterograft, comes from an animal, usually a pig. Homograft tissue, also called allograft, is skin from cadavers—deceased persons. Either of these is applied to damaged skin as a temporary cover to promote the growth of new tissue.

Burn patients, more than any others, really needed physical therapy and did receive it on the day shift. The nurses on the remaining shifts ensured that patients were given range of motion exercises, repositioning, and walks. The east wall of the unit featured a large wheel used to exercise hands and arms. Patients turned the wheel as many times as possible to strengthen their muscles and prevent contractures.

Burn Unit Patient Rounds

After I was shown around the unit, it was time for patient rounds, starting with phase one. The patient in room one was a forty-five-year-old female with second- to third-degree burns over fifty percent of her body.

CHAPTER 6 WORKING THE BURN UNIT

She had narrowly escaped a fire in her apartment. Burns near her neck and chest affected her breathing. A tracheostomy was placed (a hole through the windpipe with a breathing tube), and she was on a ventilator, which pumped air into her lungs.

Since she was on a ventilator, she received a bed bath for her personal hygiene. Even though we gave her a pain shot, she cried throughout the bath. I removed the old dressings and rinsed the wounds with saline and covered the areas with sterile towels. I quickly learned the process of soaking the fine mesh gauze in a jar of silver sulfadiazine (an antibiotic) and cutting the gauze with a blade to fit the body part and dress all of the wounds.

Room two was empty, so on to room three. This patient was a fifty-seven-year-old male who had third-degree burns over his chest from a pot of hot water. When the accident had happened, he had been working twelve hours and was very tired. He reported almost dropping the entire pot but in the process of recovering it, splashed himself.

He could be bathed in a tub. The treatment room held two bathtubs—one large with a mechanical lift and one small tub. The deeper large tub would allow soaking of the chest burns. We got him into the mechanical lift, I removed the old dressings, and we slowly submerged him into the tub. His treatment went without any incident.

Next we moved to phase two—these rooms were semi-private.

The four male patients in rooms four and five had all been in a jeep accident with a subsequent explosion. The two patients in room four were less injured, with first- and second-degree burns on about thirty-five percent of their bodies, mainly their arms and legs. The patients in room five had been in the front seats and had more intense injuries, specifically to their faces.

Nursing, Yes I Do!

The patient in room six whose bed was by the door was a seventy-five-year-old male who had tripped over his shoes, went airborne, and landed on his hands over an electric heating device.

The patient in room six, whose bed was by the window, was a sixty-nine-year-old male who was setting up to entertain a female friend and accidently lit his curtains on fire instead of a candle. He sustained burns to his arms.

One patient in room seven was a twenty-five-year-old female with healed second-degree burns to the lower body from excessively hot bath water. She was ready for discharge.

The other patient in room seven was a nineteen-year-old female with almost-healed third-degree burns to her buttocks. This girl had consumed too much alcohol and had leaned against a home heating radiator.

Room eight had one patient—a thirty-eight-year-old with almost-healed second-degree burns to her face; she had fallen asleep with a lit cigarette, which had ignited her pillow.

Laura, Fran, Marge, and I completed all the phase two patients' treatments. Most patients needed dressing changes two times per day, and we distributed those among the three shifts. It would be impossible to do all the treatments and get patients ready for surgery in one shift. It was not unusual to have two patients go for surgery in one day.

Typical surgeries for burn patients included surgical debridements (taking off the burnt skin), retrieving graft tissue from good skin to replace damaged skin, relieving pressure from contracted skin, and insertion of central lines (for IV treatments).

Fran routinely met with the trauma surgeon Dr. Bovo, as well as Dr. Freeman and Dr. Bandana, both plastic surgeons. Dr. Freeman was a hot-headed egotistical maniac. When he arrived in the unit, he demanded full attention. Dr. Bandana was much nicer and very patient. Dr. Bovo

CHAPTER 6 WORKING THE BURN UNIT

was not on our staff, but referred his burn patients from his hospital to us because they did not have such a specialized unit.

Dr. Freeman was the plastic surgeon for all the boys in the jeep accident. When he came to see the two in room five, I quickly gathered gauze pads, saline, sterile towels, and a debridement tray.

He was in his usual crabby mood. "Come on now, hurry . . . I have a lot to do today."

I whispered to myself, "Like I don't."

Fortunately, I had medicated both boys an hour before, or we would have needed earmuffs to block the screams of agony. It did not help that Dr. Freeman was not very gentle.

One the wounds were all debrided, Dr. Freeman peeled off his gloves, threw them on the floor, and left.

One of the boys looked at me. "What is his problem?"

I replied, "An overactive ego."

When I was finished the cleanup and redressed the burns for the boys in room five, I sat down to update their charts. Laura was speaking to the internists and surgeons and transcribing orders. Fran and the fire commissioner entered and made some small talk with us about a conference we would attend the next day with the fire commissioner.

At the change of shift, I met with Jackie and Janet to catch up with them and let them know how things were going. I went home feeling excited about my new position.

Wednesday was the burn conference day: The fire commissioner would teach the doctors more about burns—how they happen, why they happen, the extent of injury based on the burning agent, and so on.

I had been told to come in at 6:30 a.m., remove all the patients' dressings not done by the night shift and apply saline soaks. Vanessa and Stella were both working that day, so that made things easier. Marge helped us as well.

All the patients were ready for rounds by 8 a.m. Vanessa, Stella, and I took different patients so we could be available as needed during the rounds.

Laura and Fran walked with Dr. Bovo, Dr. Bandana, and the fire commissioner.

I leaned toward Vanessa. "Where's Dr. Freeman?"

"Oh, he hardly ever comes to these things."

After rounds, we went to the conference room, where doughnuts and coffee were waiting.

While the others met, Vanessa, Stella, Marge, and I bathed and dressed the burns on our almost-full unit. When we had finished taking care of the patients, Laura and Fran filled us in on what the fire commissioner had taught them in the conference.

Over time I grew increasingly comfortable with the routine of changing dressings and applying treatments. I was so grateful to have Marge there, as both tubs required sterilization after each use, and she did the bulk of that task. On occasion, if I hosed down the big tub, scrubbed it with the brush or did the smaller tub, I was soaked by the time I was done. It was not unusual for us to change our scrubs once or twice during a shift when busy.

If a patient had a particular infection, we would use a weak bleach in the bath water. I recall watching as the patient would step into the tub and let out an earth rattling screech—then gradually adjust and lower into the tub. Once a patient was in the tub, I did my best to clean him or her quickly and get the person to the treatment room. My supplies were always handy, and I moved swiftly to cut the fine mesh gauze impregnated with silver sulfadiazine cream, an antibiotic, to fit the burns. After dressing so many

CHAPTER 6 WORKING THE BURN UNIT

body parts, I knew just how much gauze to use for a finger, hand, arm, leg, or whatever else.

Passing meal trays for burn patients was like serving royalty. They had more food on their trays than any other patient in the hospital, as they needed, most importantly, the extra protein. High doses of vitamin C, in divided doses, were a usual part of the med regime. This was usually given orally but at times we administered it via IV. Demerol, Dilaudid, or plain morphine for pain relief was also part of the med regime for our patients.

To stabilize their electrolytes, we often gave Lactated Ringers. This is a solution of salts and other minerals that rehydrates the body and provides fuel, which helps healing. All burn patients routinely had colloid oncotic pressure blood level labs. This test monitors the fluid shift in the cardiovascular system.

Our unit, like the operating room (OR), had to maintain an environment that was as sterile as possible. When a patient was due for surgery, we would wheel him or her on a cart to the unit door and an OR tech would meet us on the other side of the door with a unit cart, minus the mattress. We would click the two carts together, then slide the mattress to the OR tech's cart, unclick the carts, and the patient would then be en route to the OR.

A New Burn Patient

New admissions would bypass the emergency room and come directly to our admitting treatment room. About four weeks into my term in the unit, I had my first new patient. We received the call from the ER that the patient was en route. Marge, Vanessa, Fran, and I prepared the room with bottles of saline, gauze, IV supplies, a cut down tray (a tray that held surgical instruments), foley catheter (for draining urine), intubation tray (supplies for putting a tube in the airway), ambu bag (for pushing air into the lungs), and oxygen.

The patient was a forty-year-old man who, while at work, touched a loose electrical connection. Not only did he have an electric burn, but he also had a heart attack.

He arrived, and first we had to establish the ABC: airway, breathing, circulation. Next, we located the entrance and exit wounds. The entrance wound was at the hand, and we found two exit wounds—one at the shoulder and the other at the foot.

"We need to watch for a brachial blow out," Fran said.

In this kind of situation, the brachial artery—the main artery in the upper arm—could literally pop open and bleed like a fountain. I hoped and prayed that would not happen, as he could die quickly from the hemorrhage.

Dr. Nemi and the new surgical resident, Dr. Ho, arrived to help assess and treat the man. With teamwork, we got the patient evaluated, treated, and admitted to his room.

What a day! I had just enough time to update the charts before Jackie and Janet came in for the second shift. My hard work and dedication to the hospital was apparently paying off, as I received another raise that brought me up to $7 an hour.

I was exhausted when I got home and had no problems sleeping.

When I arrived the next morning, Nelson the night nurse said, "The electrical burn admission—he had a brachial blowout last night."

"Oh no! Is he okay?"

"Yeah, I was at the bedside, so I tied off the bleeder with a clamp."

"Good heavens, Nelson. You saved his life!"

He shrugged. "I did what had to be done."

CHAPTER 6 WORKING THE BURN UNIT

Before he went home, everyone on the day shift thanked him for his good work.

Paperwork Versus Patient Care

The boys from the jeep fire were all improving, and we needed to work with them to improve their range of motion. They frequently used the wheel on the wall.

Laura had left the unit suddenly, and in the interim Fran took the role of head nurse. We worked together well, and she was impressed with my ability to run the unit when she had responsibilities to complete as the supervisor.

Jackie and Janet had each worked in the BTC for two and a half years to my three months, but Fran asked me to take the position of head nurse. This did not sit well with Jackie and Janet. I had to dismiss their feelings and focus on being a leader for the unit.

Since we were down one nurse, the workload was greater. I would arrive an hour early and check supplies and medications before getting the night shift report. If residents, surgeons, or consultants came in the morning, I would have to stop whatever I was doing to discuss patients' statuses, review orders, and delegate newly ordered tasks.

As far as transcribing the orders, it would wait until after lunch. "Lunch ... what is that?" I said it all too often.

Most weekdays I worked with either Vanessa or Stella, plus Marge, who was blessed to not have to work weekends. Something had happened while she had been working many years before that, and management had promised she would never have to work weekends again. I never found out any details nor did I need to know.

Fran felt confident in me, and I was happy about that, but at times I felt a little abandoned. "I really need a secretary to transcribe the orders, so treatments get done," I said.

Nursing, Yes I Do!

Fran sighed, but she nodded. "I'll try to arrange it, but I can't make any promises."

One extremely busy day, I had my period with killer cramps. I was doing a treatment on the patient in room two. She had been admitted the previous night with second- and third-degree burns to her arms, legs, and feet.

I gave her a bed bath and dressed her wounds, moving ever so slowly and trying not to show the pain in my face.

She noticed my agony. "You look worse than I feel."

I smiled, not sure how to respond to that. But then I decided to be honest. "Cramps."

"Ugh. I get it."

The desk was full of charts with orders. I reviewed them and made a list of what had to be done for treatment changes and gave it to Stella. We still had two patients to prepare for surgery, and I did that. By then it was lunchtime, and the trays and afternoon meds had to be passed.

After lunch, the first patient returned from surgery, quickly followed by the second. I checked their vital signs and dressings, as well as the post-op orders.

Stella had just finished the last morning treatment, and we had three afternoon treatments to do before 3 p.m., just two hours away.

I looked at all the paperwork waiting to be completed. *Do I leave the orders for the evening shift to transcribe or not do some of the treatments?*

My favorite supervisor, Mrs. Thorn, was out, so I called the day supervisor filling in for her. "Can you send a secretary to the burn unit? I need

CHAPTER 6 WORKING THE BURN UNIT

to focus on patient care, so without a secretary, I may have to leave the orders for the evening shift."

We did not get a secretary.

Our splash burn patient, now in phase two, had received a skin graft, a procedure wherein healthy skin is removed from one part of the body and used to cover the burn. His graft came off his thigh and was placed on his chest. After his surgery, he developed chest pain.

It was not a full code, but we did have to summon the medical staff and administer emergency medications. That took us an hour.

Stella and I met back at the nurses' station. I glanced at the clock. "One hour left to do three treatments—and transcribe orders." Fran was out of town at a burn conference, and my cramps were still killing me.

Stella and I completed the three treatments, and I had to leave the orders for Jackie and Janet. When they arrived, I gave them my report, explaining why the orders weren't done.

Wordlessly they glanced at each other and then back to me, with expressions that said, *That's of no concern to me.*

By then I was getting punchy. "If you need to report me, then do so . . . I did the best I could."

Well, they did report me. The next day, I had to meet with Fran and receive a verbal warning. "I'm uncomfortable doing this," she said, "because I know how hard you work. But it had to be done."

I nodded. "I knew that when I talked to them yesterday."

Fran gave a weak smile. "Just understand—if you should get reported again, it'll be a written warning, and a third time, a suspension."

Maybe I should have been upset. But I hoped my incident would send a message.

It did not.

We had many more days of poor staffing. I skipped meals, delayed going to the bathroom, and stayed late to transcribe orders.

Jackie and Janet knew I was working hard to complete all that needed done, and they never reported me again. After all, being the charge nurse of the unit came with the extra responsibilities.

I loved the work in the unit. Watching patients regrow their skin day by day seemed almost miraculous. But I was getting concerned about the possibility of losing my nursing license because of an error. Poor staffing is no excuse for errors, and I worked too hard for my nursing license to risk losing it over paperwork or worse, risk harming a patient.

I had been at Bastille County Hospital for three years, with both intensive care and burn treatment experience. I figured I would not have too much trouble finding a job.

It was time to look elsewhere.

Chapter 7

SEARCHING FOR NEW EMPLOYMENT

I sat down at my mother's typewriter and put together a draft resume. After going over it with her, I made the necessary changes and typed another copy on high-quality paper.

The want ads in the newspaper showed no openings in the local hospitals. Bastille had several hospitals in other areas, but Ethan and I were content in the south section of town. A job at St. Christopher's would be perfect because it was within walking distance from our apartment. But it was difficult to get hired there unless you knew someone—especially a nun.

I mentally reviewed my former colleagues and remembered that Sister Castille had left BCH to work at St. Christopher's in the emergency room.

My nerves jangled a bit as I called their unit and left my name with a request to have her call me at her convenience.

The person who had answered the phone asked, "Does she know you?"

"I'm a colleague." Which I was . . . in the not-so-distant past.

Sister Castille called me back and listened to my request. "I'm so happy to hear you're considering working at St. Christopher's! Of course, you may use me as a reference."

The next day, I walked into the human resources office with my resume and asked for an application for employment. A gruff woman with dark

Nursing, Yes I Do!

red hair and a secretarial name badge handed an application to me. "Fill it out and return it to me."

When I handed the completed form back to the secretary, she put it in a large pile.

About a week later, I received a call from St. Christopher's asking me to come in for an interview in two days at 10 a.m. That would mean a call off from my job at BCH. But of course, I told the caller, "I'll be there."

On the day of my appointment, I dressed as professionally as possible, in my navy skirt and a cream-colored blouse. I arrived at the office of the director of nurses.

"Have a seat," the secretary said. "Sister Agnes will be with you shortly."

After what felt like an eternity, I picked up a magazine to avoid staring at the secretary or just awkwardly staring into space. I glanced through the pages and found an article on a medical condition called lupus that captured my attention. I fell deep into concentration.

After a while I realized Sister Agnes was standing in front of me. I almost jumped out of my seat.

She gazed down at me in a very probing manner and said nothing.

After a painfully long silence I said, "Good morning, Sister," stood up, and shook her hand.

She then smiled. "Follow me." We walked into her office. "I reviewed your resume and found it very impressive."

"Thank you."

"I also had an opportunity to speak with Sister Castille, who praised your work at BCH."

"It was a pleasure working with Sister Castille."

"We have an opening in the intensive care unit, would you be interested?"

"Yes, very much so."

CHAPTER 7 SEARCHING FOR NEW EMPLOYMENT

"I must warn you, however"—she paused—"there is a contagious disease in their unit."

My jaw dropped open.

"Six of the staff nurses are pregnant."

I laughed. "Oh, how nice."

"There is a rumor something may be in the water."

"Not a bad disease to get." I smiled.

She finally laughed. "When can you start?"

"I will need to give two weeks' notice to my current employer."

"That's acceptable." She scheduled my orientation and asked that I bring in my current vaccination record. "I can offer you $8 an hour."

"That will be perfect, thank you."

Fastest interview I ever had.

I called Cassie to tell her about the new job.

"Oh, Aubrey, that's wonderful! I'm so happy for you."

"Thanks. And how are things going for you?"

"I'm getting a promotion to full-time evening supervisor."

"That's great, but aren't you leaving soon?" My friend's impending departure weighed down my joy.

"Yes, it's a temporary role. We're leaving for San Francisco within the next six months."

My last two weeks at BCH passed quickly. Jackie would take position on days as the new charge nurse, and Janet would stay on evenings for a while to train two new nurses. Eventually she would also move to the day shift.

On my last day, Fran brought in a cake, and we cut it at the change of shift so Jackie and Janet could have a slice and say their farewells. Their goodbyes were genuinely heartfelt, and they wished me well.

Starting at St Christopher's

General orientation at St. Christopher's included staff, nurses, aides, clerical workers, and housekeepers. On the first day of orientation, in addition to a tour, we reviewed the hospital's policies and safety measures. I buddied up with two girls. Toni, also assigned to the ICU, was an extremely attractive lady a little older than I with short blonde hair. She appeared fearless of anything that came her way. Kathy would work in the business office and was also attractive—much younger than I was, with beautiful long dark brown hair. I shared my story of my interview and the contagious disease of pregnancy, as that created a great ice breaker.

The hospital had two sections—one had been built about fifty years earlier and the other had just been built the previous year. The old section featured five floors, and the new section held eight floors. The hospital had moved all the patients out of the old section and into the new one, so the older part of the building could be used for offices and clinics. Since this was a Catholic hospital, it had a chapel—much larger than the one at BCH.

On day two of orientation, all the nurses were expected to complete a separate training and take a test on medical surgical nursing. *Ugh, a test.* Thankfully, I passed.

On day three the ICU nurses received separate training, so that session was just for Toni and me. This day was more intense and involved training primarily on medications, IVs, and mechanical ventilators. We had two instructors. Abigal was a matronly woman with tightly curled black hair and wore her nurse's cap perfectly in the center back of her head. She went over the medications and IVs. Sarah was tall, thin, and stately. She went over the ventilators. We had no written test, but we spent the last forty-five minutes on answering oral questions from the instructors. Toni and I pretty much shared answering questions and did so correctly, with just a couple of mistakes by each of us.

CHAPTER 7 SEARCHING FOR NEW EMPLOYMENT

When orientation day four came, Toni and I were to start in the unit and work with Sarah for the day.

Sarah showed us around. "When we moved over here from the old building, they combined the medical ICU and surgical ICU. We were supposed to have six medical beds on one side and six surgical beds on the other side." She waved a hand at either side of the floor. "That didn't work, because we have no control over how many medical or surgical patients we have."

I nodded. That made sense.

"The new unit's been open for about seven months." She paused in her stroll down the hall and leaned close, her voice low. "I must admit, for about the first three months or so, the nurses from the different sides did *not* have a good relationship with each other *at all*." She rolled her eyes toward the ceiling. "Outbursts, confrontations, you name it. The supervisors had to intervene a few times."

"What did they fight over?" I was glad she was confiding in us, but wary about what I had gotten myself into.

"Usually, differences in how each of the units is run." Sarah glanced around as if to make sure no one was listening. "Things are getting better. The head nurse has her hands full, but she had a good handle on the situation." She pushed open a door and led us into a conference room.

There we received a report from the head nurse, Anne. We were assigned one patient each.

My patient was a seventy-five-year-old woman with chronic obstructive lung disease as well as hypertension and a sixty-year history of smoking one-half pack of cigarettes per day. Her doctors had been trying to convince her to stop smoking because her lungs had been failing for the last fifteen years—but she refused.

She had collapsed at home and turned cyanotic (a bluish skin discoloration caused by low blood oxygen). Fortunately, her son was a

Nursing, Yes I Do!

paramedic, and he did CPR until the ambulance came and transported her to St. Christopher's.

By the time I was her nurse, she had been intubated and was on a mechanical ventilator to help her breathe. A central IV line was inserted in her chest via the subclavian vein (which runs under the clavicle and connects to the jugular vein in the throat), and she had a foley catheter to drain her bladder. Sarah spent a lot of time going over the ventilator, explaining assist control pressures and tidal volume.

My patient was weak, but she was alert to her surroundings and could follow simple commands. I learned quickly how to communicate with an intubated patient to meet the person's needs. We were instructed to use a magic slate or interpret the eye and body movements. Sarah alternated between Toni and me, helping with bathing the patient and changing sheets.

The morning flew. At lunchtime, the cafeteria was packed with workers and visitors. In those days, smoking was still allowed indoors, with no separation from nonsmokers. Many of the nurses and physicians at St. Christopher's had that nasty habit.

The food was palatable at best, but when you were hungry, it would do. Toni, Sarah, and I talked all through lunch, discussing patient care and medical conditions, being discreet and not mentioning anything that would identify our patients.

The day shift was allowed a thirty-minute break in the morning and a thirty-minute lunch. Since we had been training all morning, we spent the whole hour at lunch. The evening and night shifts each took one sixty-minute meal break.

Then it was time for us to get back to the unit.

We spent the afternoon reviewing the doctor's orders and carrying them out. Thank heaven, no more transcribing orders! We had a secretary—or ward clerk, as they were called—for each side. Wanda and Iris were our ward clerks and lifesavers.

CHAPTER 7 SEARCHING FOR NEW EMPLOYMENT

Toni and I worked with Sarah the next day as well, and by the day after that, we were on our own—but of course Sarah was there every day as the pulmonary specialist and was a great resource.

Full-timers like Toni and me were expected to work any of three shifts, and at times, you might end up doubling back, like working a night shift and then second shift the following day. That was a killer.

Our aides were great. My greatest challenge was getting to know my female coworkers, learning their personalities and what buttons not to push. I was twenty-three years old and in the same age group as most of the girls in the unit.

The second- and third-shift part-time nurses were primarily women in their thirties to forties with children, and they worked around spouses' schedules to be there for the children.

We had a few part-time nurses who were graduates of a three-year program the hospital had run at one time. They received special privilege working hours during their childbearing years, and that had never changed, even though by this time they were all grandmothers. They worked 9 a.m. to 3 p.m., and no weekends or holidays.

Speaking of childbearing, we heard Brahms' "Lullaby" over the intercom every time a baby was born in the obstetric unit. No matter where you were in the hospital, people always smiled when it played.

Transportation

I often walked to work, even when I worked an evening shift. I would ask for a ride home from a coworker, or Ethan would pick me up. After three months, it was time to get a second car. Since our primary car was a used one, we invested in a new one—a Buick Regal, golden brown in color; what a beauty.

Ethan and I took the Regal to Detroit to visit his brother and sister-in-law. We left the old car in his mom's driveway so his other brother could use it while we were away. When we arrived home and picked up the old car, Ethan took the old one while I drove the Regal home.

As I pulled out of the driveway, something fell off. The steering wheel became difficult to turn, as if it were fighting against me. My muscles tugged as if I were lifting lead weights. I had to use all my strength just to turn the wheel. It was only a ten-minute drive, but it felt like hours. I was a nervous wreck the whole time. *What is wrong with this car?*

By the time I pulled into our own driveway, I was dripping sweat. It turned out that our power steering belt had snapped. Thank heaven it did not happen on the highway.

Settled into ICU Routines

When I worked days, I went in early, had coffee, and talked to whomever I knew in the cafeteria. I frequently saw Janice, who had a cigarette and coffee then as well as later during her morning break. She did eat lunch but always snuck in that cigarette.

Since the unit had six beds on each side, Anne, the head nurse, assigned a team leader for each side, and then the team leader scheduled patient assignments and breaks. Anne and Abigal worked closely together to ensure that everything flowed smoothly.

On day shift, the team leader made the assignments for her two nurses and two aides. The team leader was responsible for doing rounds with the head nurse and the doctors, reviewing orders, and to pass medications. The other nurses assisted the aides with bathing, administered treatments, and monitored IVs, among other tasks. One particular aide we all appreciated was Janelle. She was our "work mother" who was both compassionate during our time of need and critical when she felt we needed to be disciplined.

CHAPTER 7 SEARCHING FOR NEW EMPLOYMENT

On evening and night shift, there was one team leader, one nurse, and one aide for each side. On occasional days, when we had more critical patients, we were allowed an extra nurse.

Because we had to make sure there was sufficient coverage in the unit around break times, we had three scheduled morning break times and three lunch times for days—and two each for the evening and night shifts.

Since these patients were so critically ill, it was not unusual for medication doses to require mathematical calculations. I would check my math a couple times to make sure it was correct.

Most of the patients were on ventilators to aide their breathing, had central lines for IV fluids and medications, and had foley catheters to drain their bladders and monitor their urine output.

Blood tests via the artery in the wrist, inner elbow, or groin were also routine for ventilator patients, as this would show how well their blood was oxygenated. Blood samples from an artery provided insight on the condition of the lungs and the body's ability to compensate by balancing the Ph level. A normal Ph is 7.35–7.45. A low Ph level reveals acidosis (excess acid) and a high Ph reveals alkalosis (excess alkali). The blood sample measures the Ph, oxygen, carbon dioxide, bicarbonate, and base levels. This test is essential for patients with respiratory problems. Sarah signed me off on performing arterial blood gases two weeks after I started.

Lidocaine drips were ordered on patients with irregular heart rhythms and were placed on a pump, scheduling a precise drip rate. Nipride was given to patients with sky-high blood pressures, while on the flipside, dopamine was for those struggling with low blood pressure.

Respiratory therapists frequently ensured the ventilators were cleaned and that settings remained accurate. I became remarkably close with all of them.

The lab techs were in usually before day shift, doing routine morning labs. Now that I was doing arterial blood draws, it came in handy if the lab tech could not get a blood sample via the vein and the patient was also due for an arterial blood gas—ABG as we most often called it. I could obtain all the samples via the ABG . . . with a doctor's order, of course.

Probably the most challenging cases were head and neck injuries. Patients who had a head injury and additional pressure in the brain from fluid, had an intracranial pressure or ICP catheter to measure the pressure in the brain. We had to reposition these patients in bed ever so carefully, so as not to disrupt the catheter in their brain.

Patients with neck injuries might have a device to stabilize the head known as a Crutchfield Tong or Halo Traction. These patients also had to be turned ever so carefully. They were placed either on a Stryker Frame bed or Circo-Electric bed. The former was like a stretcher with two mattresses, one for the supine (face up) position and the other for the prone (face down) position. You literally had to lock the top and bottom of the stretcher, and with one nurse or aide at the head of the bed and one at the foot, quickly turn the patient over 180 degrees.

The Circo-Electric bed had two stretcher mattresses with 360-degree circular bars on either side of the bed that would slowly turn the patient from supine to prone and vice versa. Patients were rotated every two hours.

When you worked in this environment, you could not be ill. I came in one day with an upset stomach and then developed diarrhea. You were lucky if you could get to the bathroom to pee, let alone have the runs. Quickly, I went to the satellite pharmacy on site and asked for anything available. I was given a basic, over-the-counter anti-diarrheal. Fortunately, it worked quickly, and I could complete my shift.

The residents in the unit were around our age and flirted a lot with the nurses. I would just smile and be grateful that I no longer had any dating concerns. The attending physicians who were older were much more respectful.

CHAPTER 7 SEARCHING FOR NEW EMPLOYMENT

One day, when I was giving my oral report to the evening shift nurses, Toni and Christine, my timing was apparently not good. I was sitting between them, giving the report, and before I knew it, the two of them were standing and yelling at each other over my head.

Toni blurts out, "Since Alex is off today, maybe you will get your work done today and I won't have to finish it for you."

Christine drops her jaw and follows with, "How dare you, Alex and I have a great relationship, which is more than I can say for you since your two divorces."

I looked up at them. "Whoa! I would like to go home, so can you please sit down so I can give you the report?"

They did and were quiet for the remaining report time.

I just chuckled as I left the unit.

I will not forget the time an aide, Roxie, caused a contemptible uproar for me. Roxie was an aide who loved to gossip. On busy days, we often missed a morning break. If that happened and we were scheduled for the third morning break slot, we could ask the team leader to let us go on the first lunch slot. No big deal.

I had a hectic morning one day when I was scheduled for the third morning break, so I switched my lunch break from third to first slot. Roxie told the nurse I was originally scheduled to share morning break with that I didn't want to go with her, so I missed my break on purpose.

I explained to the nurse that Roxie's story was untrue. At first, she didn't believe me, but after she learned about other instances when Roxie had done this, she came around.

We both sighed and said, "Roxie, Roxie, Roxie."

Losses

Sometimes patients died in the unit—whether it was an unsuccessful resuscitation or a decision by the family to remove artificial means and

Nursing, Yes I Do!

allow a peaceful death. Whether or not a patient or family was Catholic, we always offered pastoral care that respected their religious practice.

My first experience in removing a patient from artificial means involved a seventy-nine-year-old male with multiple medical conditions. He had been declining daily, as shown by his blood work, urine output, and responses.

I was working evening shift that day, and it was my first shift with him, so I hadn't developed a relationship with him or his family. This may have made it easier.

Day shift had already spent time with the family, so my part was to meet with the doctor, family, respiratory therapy, and pastoral care in the room.

The doctor met me in the hallway. "He's in full organ shut down and experiencing extreme pain."

I bit my lip and nodded.

He pushed open the door. Inside the room I saw the patient's family: his wife with their daughter and son-in-law. The doctor gave the family a few more kind words of wisdom. Then he gave me the nod to discontinue the ventilator.

I pressed down the power button turning off the ventilator and extracted the man's breathing tube.

The patient had only two gasps for air, and then he peacefully drifted off.

The doctor had his stethoscope ready. He listened for a heartbeat and breathing. He heard none. "Time of death, 4:05 p.m."

The family wept quietly, and I consoled the wife primarily, as the son-in-law consoled the daughter.

It is never easy to lose a patient, but it does get easier, knowing how to care for the family.

CHAPTER 7 SEARCHING FOR NEW EMPLOYMENT

Patients in the unit spanned various ages. One was a twenty-five-year-old woman—so close to my own age—brought in with a head injury from an unknown trauma. She had been admitted the night before, so by the time I came in she was already intubated, on a ventilator, and had multiple IVs.

She was nonresponsive and surrounded by many family members. A certain chill filled the air, metaphorically. I felt the tension among some family members.

Around mid-morning, I overhead one family member say to another "It was her husband's fault."

Shortly after that, a police officer arrived and ushered the husband out of the unit.

Something is wrong here.

I carried on with my work on my twenty-five-year-old, as well as my other patient, being as professional as I could.

When I returned the next day, my twenty-five-year-old patient remained in critical condition. The night shift had taken her to surgery to evacuate bleeding in her brain. She was not responding, even to deep pain stimuli. Her doctor ordered an electroencephalogram (EEG)—a test that measures electrical activity in the brain.

There was none.

The following day, she again was not responsive to deep pain stimuli, so another EEG was done. Still no brain activity.

Her husband was back; he only spoke to the doctor, not to other family members.

The patient's sister was the only one who occasionally asked me how her sister was doing. I had never dealt with a group of people who were obviously so torn and had so little communication, not only among themselves but also with me or any of the other nursing staff.

Nursing, Yes I Do!

Occasionally each of us would reach out to them by offering to bring water, or to sit with them, or to answer any questions they might have, but they declined.

I grew very tense in that room.

The following day, I witnessed the discussion between the husband and the doctor about removing the patient from the ventilator and initiating euthanasia—allowing the patient to die painlessly.

The other family members were brought in from the waiting room.

Anne told me the husband had signed the consent to remove all artificial means of support. Since this was my patient, I would stop the ventilator after Sister Joel had prayed with the family.

I had turned off ventilators for other patients a few times before, but this was different.

A family member hissed at the husband, "This is your fault."

Once Sister Joel started her customary prayer, my eyes began to swell. I felt tears building, ready to burst out, so I hurried out of the room to our nurse's lounge and cried in there. I was overwhelmed with emotions including concerns of the family discontent with each other and her impending death at such a young age.

Anne came into the lounge a couple minutes later and grabbed my shoulders. "Get yourself together."

I just kept whimpering, "I am trying; just give me a few minutes." I had made a fool of myself, but I was most concerned not to upset the family.

She put her arms around me. "I know this is a tough one."

Her compassion almost made me cry harder. I so appreciated her understanding.

"I took her off the vent," Anne said. "It's all over." She agreed that I could wait to finish my work in the room until after the family left. "I'll send someone in to tell you when it's time," she said.

I scrubbed away my tears with the sleeve of my blouse. "Thank you."

CHAPTER 7 SEARCHING FOR NEW EMPLOYMENT

Later on, Iris, one of the ward clerks, let me know the family was gone. "Are you okay?" she added.

"Yeah. I'll be fine." But when I finally stepped out into the unit again, I felt emotionally numb from this stressful situation.

Chapter 8
MORE ABOUT THE STAFF

I grew close with three other RNs. Mallory and Carrie were the same age as I, and Brandy was a year younger. None of them were married. We enjoyed the time if we were scheduled to work together on the same side, and we could ask each other questions without feeling embarrassed.

The residents in this hospital behaved better than those at BCH. Someone must have put the fear of God into them! Workplace culture really is important to foster an environment where people can thrive.

Some residents were easy to work with—others not so much. Since they were so close to our age, we called them by their first name. Sam and Alex were the docs in demand by the young unattached nurses. They were both very handsome, as well as being personable and good doctors. Phil was a stately fellow, who was serious and knew his stuff. Gary was cheerful and amiable, which at times overshadowed his intelligence.

Residents are doctors who have completed medical school but haven't yet passed their board exams. You may have heard first-year residents are called *interns*. Residents work under the supervision of board-certified doctors, who attend their rounds with them and are therefore called *attending physicians* or *attendings* for short.

As for the attending doctors at St. Christopher's, I had a few favorites. Dr. Castaldo was the pulmonologist and medical director of the unit. He and Sarah worked together regularly. He was a kind, soft spoken, attractive

CHAPTER 8 MORE ABOUT THE STAFF

man who really knew pulmonology. Understanding how to interpret arterial blood gases is difficult, and he explained it well.

Dr. Parks was a diabetic specialist and knew her patients extremely well. I marveled at the way she would order insulin coverage and teach her patients how to eat correctly. She even gave each of her patients a chart to use if they ate at various chain restaurants, so they knew what to order within their diabetic diet. They did well and had only short stays in the unit and no complications. Problems only arose when they went home and did not follow her instructions. Her patients probably needed to take her home with them. She was a tiny thing, but when she spoke, you listened.

One patient of hers had a complicated case of diabetes, and we adjusted his meds about every two hours. Dr. Parks slept in the respite room overnight and asked to be awakened if his blood sugar changed outside the expected range. Fortunately, the next morning, the patient stabilized and was transferred to a medical floor.

Dr. Green was a general surgeon, and I remember the day he was on call for emergency surgeries. A male child was brought into our emergency room (ER) from a motor vehicle accident. He was barely responsive, and his belly was hard and obviously bleeding internally. Dr. Green called for equipment to open the child's belly so he could tie off the bleeding vessel. Everyone in the ER said he couldn't do it there and must wait for an operating room.

"The child will be dead by that time!" Dr. Green demanded the equipment. "Would you prefer to be responsible for his death?"

A nurse rushed to get the necessary equipment.

On the nurse's return, another nurse joined him, and the procedure was done in the ER. The child's life was saved.

In the ICU, Dr. Green was extremely respected and for good reasons, based on that case and others that happened in the unit. His response time was immediate, and his surgical technique was flawless.

Let us not forget the hospital chaplains. On a chilly February afternoon at the start of my shift, our hospital chaplain asked if we nurses wished to have our *throats* blessed.

As a Catholic, I followed the traditions of the church but didn't fully understand them all. I suppose I had blind faith.

Caring For the Obese

The chronically ill patients we cared for in the ICU were often overweight by at least forty pounds due to inactivity secondary to their illnesses. Nurses build strong muscles in their arms, abdomen, and legs, especially when they use correct body mechanics and maintain healthy activity levels outside of work.

Nevertheless, you can still hurt yourself, and in our ICU this happened often. In the early 1980s, back belts were just starting to be used, and they were optional. If you did use one, it was crucial to wear the back belt correctly. I bought one and used it only when I had an excessively obese patient.

I recall one patient who was 608 pounds. I'll call her Darcie. She had called a cab to take her to the doctor's office because she was short of breath. As she walked down her front stairs to the waiting cab, she slipped on the ice and fell. She was still alert, oriented, and breathing but with difficulty. The cab driver immediately called 911.

When the ambulance arrived, they knew Darcie would not fit on a gurney. Fortunately, firefighters had also responded. It took six men to lift her and place her on the floor of the ambulance.

When she arrived at the hospital, they placed her on two gurneys that were securely tied together and evaluated her in the ER. Her vital signs revealed a temperature of 101 degrees Fahrenheit (high), a pulse of 112 (fast), respirations at 40 per minute (very fast), and blood pressure of 140 over 70 (not too far off normal).

CHAPTER 8 MORE ABOUT THE STAFF

Darcie was able to answer questions and gave permission for the staff to draw labs, do an electrocardiogram, take chest Xrays, and give her oxygen to help her breathe.

With the utmost professionalism, the staff undressed her and placed an oversized hospital gown over her. She could not get her arms through the sleeves.

The head nurse of the ER called the director of nursing (DON) and asked if larger gowns were available or if a seamstress was available to sew two gowns together. Our DON said her team would ask one of the nuns in the convent to modify some hospital gowns for Darcie.

The emergency room phoned us so we could prepare for her. We called in the maintenance crew, and they securely tied two beds together and locked them in place.

When Darcie arrived in the ICU from emergency, she was accompanied by the assigned ICU resident, one ER nurse, an aide, and three maintenance men. She was my patient, so I approached the room. Anne, Sarah, and Brandy joined me to provide extra help.

Six people were already in the room transferring her to the modified bed, so we stood at the door, watching. They got her settled.

As the maintenance men left the room, one said sternly, "Do not call us again to position this patient."

I responded, "How rude!"

I had already received a report about the patient, so as the ER staff left, the four of us entered the room and introduced ourselves to her.

Anne spoke up first. "Sarah and Brandy and I will connect you to the heart monitor and oxygen, and we'll check your catheter. Aubrey, will you please complete the admission questionnaire?" I did this while the others went about their tasks.

Once we were finished, we repositioned her and gave her a blanket, as she was cold.

Nursing, Yes I Do!

We walked out to the corridor, where Anne looked me in the eye, her voice firm. "Do not try to reposition her without at least four people or boost without six."

I nodded.

The next day, Darcie, in room six, was my patient again. The day started out crazily, because two patients were unstable and the physicians, respiratory therapists, and nurses were running in and out of those two rooms. My two patients were stable; however, I did have to give Darcie a bed bath. First, I checked on my other patient, in room four, and gave him his medications and changed his IV bag.

As I entered room six, I greeted Daricie. "How are you today?"

She replied in a whisper. "Much better today, thank you."

She still had a slight fever and elevated heart rate and respirations, but her vitals were improved from the day before.

I procrastinated in giving her a bath because everyone was too busy to help. But by 11 a.m., I asked my nurse aide, Nancy, to meet me in the room in ten minutes.

"Sure," she said, "but we cannot lift her."

"We'll get help," I snapped. "Sorry. I didn't mean to sound punchy."

Nancy waved this off. "No problem."

I went into Darcie's room. "I'm going to start your bath."

She stared at me. "By yourself?"

"I'm confident I can wash the front of you, and we'll assess your ability to roll to your side, and then I can wash your backside."

When I wrapped her arm over her chest and bent her top leg over the bottom leg, she rolled like a ball and grabbed the side rail. Quickly I washed that side and repeated this roll to the other side to complete her bathing.

When I was done, Nancy walked in.

I packed up my supplies. "I'm done."

Nancy's jaw dropped open.

CHAPTER 8 MORE ABOUT THE STAFF

"Can you please round up four more people?" I asked. "Start with Anne."

Within three minutes, five people entered the room, and we boosted Darcie up and placed her in a comfortable position.

After five days, we were able to discharge Darcie. She went straight home from the ICU, though she was referred for home care.

One year later, she came in to visit us, 120 pounds lighter. "I still have a long way to go," she said. We all gave her a hug.

Change of Shifts

After I had worked swing shift for about eight months, word got out that staff would start working consistent shifts.

Anne handed out the sign-up forms "You can all to apply for whatever shift you want, but there's no guarantee you'll get it."

I wanted days, but if necessary, I would take evenings. I just prayed to God I would not get night shift.

"I hope I can get a day shift," said one of the part-time nurses.

"Please, God," said another. "I have to work while the kids are in school; otherwise, I have to pay for a babysitter."

We had a large pool of part-time nurses, and from their murmurings, I gather most of them felt the same way, although some would also prefer nights, when spouses could watch the kids. Even back then, the cost of childcare could be prohibitive.

The final list came out, and I did get day shift. Almost all of us on day shift were full-time. That is best, because it's the primary time the physicians come in and when surgeries or other procedures were done. Evening and night shift maintained the patients. But I can say, however, having worked many evening and night shifts, plenty of emergencies and new admissions could happen after hours.

A nurse always hopes his or her patients will be stable, but that doesn't always happen. On a quiet evening or night shift, you could pre-pour your meds for the shift. On a busy one, you were lucky if you could pass them out on time.

A procedure often done on day shift was inserting a Swan Ganz catheter. This was inserted into the heart via a vein in the upper chest or neck to measure blood flow and pressure in the heart. In the ICU, it could be done at the bedside. We were all instructed in this procedure. I brought the directions home and read them three times before I felt comfortable with it. I remember setting up for my first one and feeling nervous and grateful for help from Paula, who filled in as head nurse when Anne was off.

The second time was much easier.

By the next time a patient needed a Sawn Ganz, the directions had changed, and none of the nursing staff had been retrained . . . only the medical staff. Paula, Anne, and I hustled to assist Sam with his procedure. Thankfully, he was understanding and patient.

As much as we moved from shift to shift, patients moved in and out of the unit. Giving the day's report to the floor nurses was always entertaining. We sometimes heard comments from them like, "Oh here come those stuck-up ICU nurses," when they thought we were not in earshot.

When it was time for my review, I received a raise of twenty-five cents per hour, bringing me to $8.25 an hour.

Holidays

A week before Christmas, I learned I would work the day shift on Christmas Day and the evening shift on New Year's Day.

"Is that gonna work?" Ethan asked.

"Yeah, no problem." I jotted notes in my calendar. "I only have to prepare a side to take to Mom's for Christmas dinner by 4:30 p.m. and a dish of cookies to take to your parents' house by around 8 p.m."

He shook his head. "That's gonna make for a hectic day."

"Honey . . . all my days are hectic."

CHAPTER 8 MORE ABOUT THE STAFF

On the Friday before Christmas, the hospital held a dinner, which ran from 1–5 p.m. to allow enough time for all the staff to attend. The cafeteria was decorated nicely, and the food was so-so, but still very much appreciated.

As I ate, I thought about the evening. I'd have to swing home to pick up the food, then head to Mom's house, then to my in-laws' before getting back home to rest. Ethan was right; it would be a long and busy evening.

So, after finishing my meal, I visited the chapel. The last time I had been there was about twelve years earlier, when my dad had been a patient in that hospital.

I walked across the waiting room en route to the chapel, looking down at the star design on the flooring and remembering the times my sister and I sat in the same waiting room when our dad was a patient. We had often walked around the star just to keep ourselves busy between drawing in our coloring books. I felt the urge to walk around the star now, but resisted, afraid I'd be embarrassed if I were seen.

As I entered the chapel, I had the sensation of repose. I sat there for about fifteen minutes and just let my mind wander to a peaceful place. A little respite before all the holiday running around.

The chaplain, Father Joe, walked up and startled me. "Sorry. Is everything all right?"

I smiled, "Oh yes, Father. Just enjoying the solitude."

He chuckled. "That happens a lot in here."

Presenting a Proposal

I had been doing my own research on primary care versus team nursing for patient care. Since about 1950, most hospitals had used team nursing, but by 1981, primary care nursing was catching on.

In team nursing, a group of nurses will care for a group of patients, so each patient may receive care from different nurses each day. By contrast, in the primary care model, each patient is assigned to one main nurse who

Nursing, Yes I Do!

provides all of his or her care during the day shift, although other nurses and aides will help. In team nursing, a patient is followed by one nurse who communicates with the physician, another nurse who administers the medications, and another nurse who completes any tasks.

The main advantage to primary care nursing is that one nurse is responsible to oversee the patient's care, thereby providing greater continuity. The nurse also can develop a close relationship with the patient and the family, which improves communication. And familiarity increases the likelihood of the nurse noticing changes in the patient's condition.

The best settings for primary care are places where patients receive intense treatment for a long time, which is why intensive care units are among the places this model works well. Some hospitals employed primary care not only in these units but also on regular floors.

I brought my findings to Carrie, Mallory, and Brandy and asked if they were willing to help me make a proposal to management. They agreed.

We had after-work meetings to compile our proposal. We put together a rough draft, and Mallory, who had graduated Magna Cum Laude from her school, did the final review and made revisions. Carrie owned a typewriter, so she typed the final copy.

When we presented our final proposal to Anne, our head nurse, she was extremely impressed. We agreed that I would call Sister Frances and arrange a meeting with Carrie, Mallory, Brandy, Anne, and myself.

A few days later we met with Sister Frances in a cold, stark conference room.

Carrie, Mallory, Brandy, and I took turns making our points. The entire time we were speaking, Sister Frances kept looking at Anne.

When we finished our presentation, Sister Frances said to Anne, "Do you really think this will work here?"

I held my breath.

Anne replied, "Yes."

CHAPTER 8 MORE ABOUT THE STAFF

My relief came out like a sigh. "The four of us would like to visit a few hospitals that are already using this system to complete our research. Would that be okay?"

Sister Frances nodded. "You have one day."

We decided to go in pairs, with two of us going to one hospital and two to another, gathering data. Then we'd complete a pros and cons write up. Carrie and Mallory made an appointment with St. Christopher's North, while Brandy and I went to City Hospital.

When we arrived at City Hospital, we were directed to the second floor surgical ICU. As we entered the unit, we saw doctors and staff running to a room where a code had just been called. We saw them perform open cardiac massage and learned it was a new post-op patient experiencing complications.

Brandy and I just looked at each other. "That is something we would not see at St. Christopher's," she said.

We waited while they finished, and then the head nurse had a conference with the doctor. When the doctor left, she greeted us with a smile and ushered us into her office. "So, your unit still has team nursing, huh?"

I nodded. "Yes, we do."

"What can I do to help with your transition?"

I opened my notepad and took out a pen. We interviewed her for about two hours, learning how long they had used the new method, why they had changed, and the obstacles they had encountered. Brandy suggested we observe their process for scheduling assignments, and the criteria they used.

After we left, we stopped for lunch before heading back to put together our report for Sister Frances.

The next morning, all four of us were scheduled to work, and we had a few minutes before shift to talk about our experiences. We handed over our written reports to Anne first, and she reviewed them with Sarah, the pulmonary specialist. Then the two of them went to see Sister Frances.

At the end of the day, Anne and Sarah called all four of us into the conference room. "Sister Frances is willing to pilot this."

I kept a straight face, though I wanted to cheer.

"I think the fact that St. Christopher's North is doing primary care nursing on *all* floors and units was a big factor in her decision," Anne said.

We left the conference room buzzing with excitement, but when we mentioned the pilot to a few old timers, they just shook their heads. "It will never work."

I did not respond.

Piloting the Project

The day came to launch the primary care pilot program. When the day shift came in, Anne had already prepared the patient assignments, since she always arrived early. The day shift received an oral report from the night shift. Each nurse was responsible for one to three patients, depending on patient status and treatment needs. Two aides were available, one for each side of the unit.

When the doctors came in for rounds, they were immediately impressed that they could speak to one nurse who knew everything about the patient—even how the patient reacted to turning and positioning.

It was a hit.

St. Christopher's Hospital published its own newsletter, so Brandy, Carrie, Mallory, and I were excited to see a write-up. The following week we were all working the day the newsletter came out. Eagerly, we scanned the document and found the article. It read, in part, *"With special thanks to Sarah and the hospital administration, primary care nursing has been initiated in the ICU."*

Our mouths dropped open. We were speechless. Sarah saw our expressions and approached us. "I had no idea they were going to

CHAPTER 8 MORE ABOUT THE STAFF

write that," she said. "They know and I know the four of you did all of the work."

We thanked her for her humble response.

I Got the Disease

Ethan and I were married at age twenty-one, and because we wanted to wait a couple of years before having children, I had an intrauterine device.

By 1981, we had been married two years, and as recommended at the time, I had the IUD removed.

After the doctor removed the device, he paused. "Did you want another one?"

"Not right now. We want to consider having children for a while."

He nodded and pulled off his exam gloves.

Three weeks later, I couldn't finish my breakfast.

"Are you okay?" Ethan asked.

"Probably. I've just noticed that lately I feel nauseated a lot."

He grinned but didn't say anything.

"Fortunately, I haven't been full-on vomiting." I drank some coffee, but that didn't sit well, either. "I just feel queasy at times."

My period was due and did not arrive. So, I made an appointment with my doctor.

When I told Ethan the date of the appointment, he pulled out his calendar and frowned. "We were going to go see that house that day." We had been searching for a new home for some time and had finally found a likely possibility.

"Oh, right. What time?" I took out my calendar too, and we agreed that I would meet him at the house after my appointment.

At the doctor's office, the pregnancy test came back positive. I was ecstatic. I drove to the house as if I were flying. I could not stop smiling.

Nursing, Yes I Do!

When I arrived, Ethan was standing in the parlor with his dad and my dad. I knew my face was beaming. I focused on Ethan. "We're having a baby!"

This led to cheers, hugs, and kisses all around.

I would need to cut down to part time after the baby was born, but I was ready for that and eager to be a mom. Back home, Ethan and I sat at the kitchen table with our calendars open.

"I can continue to work full time until about my eighth month."

His brow furrowed. "Is that safe?"

"Yes, I'm confident that I'm healthy enough and strong enough to do it." My due date was about the second week of November.

Ethan wrote it in his planner. "So, I guess you'll get Thanksgiving and Christmas off this year?"

"Ha! Yes."

I needed maternity clothes, and the ones I found in the stores were not good. I began sewing like crazy.

Work clothes were no problem. We wore scrubs and had a variety of sizes available, so we had no problem finding ones to fit as our bellies grew.

Yes, we. Four other nurses all announced pregnancies within three months of each other. Baby showers were planned for all the new moms. The girls in the ICU gave me a wonderful baby shower. One of my most favorite gifts from the girls was a long, cozy navy-blue robe that I used for years.

One day, a code nine was called, and three of us pregnant nurses responded to the patient.. In the Intensive Care Unit, we generally run the code and the team assists us. In this situation, from the outside looking in, the sight of three women with big round bellies dashing all around the patient must have been pretty comical.

By the way, the patient did survive.

CHAPTER 8 MORE ABOUT THE STAFF

By the second week of October, I was waddling everywhere. I did tire easily; by the end of a shift, my back was killing me, and my legs felt like lead weights. The doctor agreed that I needed to spend less time on my feet.

I met with Anne. "I can work two more weeks, but then I'll need to take leave."

"You know, you work in a hospital. We could wheel you down to delivery if we need to."

I laughed. "Thanks, but I think I'll follow my doctor's advice."

When the day came, I did deliver our baby at St. Christopher's. It was a long labor of sixteen hours, but everyone was great to me, and our baby arrived safely.

My co-workers sneaked down to see me and our beautiful little boy, Cameron. The head nurse of the postpartum unit was like a drill sergeant—if she caught nurses from other units coming in to see their coworkers, she escorted them out, because only family were allowed to visit. She would actually stand at the center staircase and point her finger at them. "Get back to work, girls!"

In postpartum, I shared a room with a nice young girl who had also given birth to her first child.

That first night, a staff nurse asked, "Do you want a sleeping pill?"

I had never taken one before, but since I did feel a little on edge and sore, I took the pill. After a quick sitz bath, I hit the pillow like a rock.

The following day, my roommate and I had a grand old time talking the day away between feeding our little ones and receiving visitors. But that night, while I was making my last bathroom trip, my roommate screamed, "I can't breathe!"

Nursing, Yes I Do!

I ran out of the bathroom.

She was clenching her neck.

I was confused about what to do. Her coloring was still good. "I'll get a nurse." I jabbed the call button and ran to the nurses' station.

It was empty. I found no one in the recovery room either. I ran back to our room, prepared to pull the code cord.

When I got back, my roommate was sitting up and breathing, deeply and fully. She was calm, and her color was good.

"Are you okay now? I asked.

"Yeah. Probably just a panic attack."

A nurse popped into the room then and did a complete assessment on my roommate.

Exhausted by the stress and running around, I fell deeply asleep, no pills needed.

Chapter 9
EVENING SHIFTS

Christmas 1981 was fast approaching. Although I was still on maternity leave, the cardiologists invited me to their party. I was excited to go. Being a new mom, my fun time was limited, and although I had stayed in touch with Brandy, Carrie, and Mallory, I hadn't seen them much. They spent a lot of time together, as none of them were married, but Mallory was newly engaged.

The girls and I planned to go to the party together. I drove; however, we should have chosen someone else. I have a terrible internal compass and needed much guidance to get there. We did finally arrive safely.

The party was held at their office, with about one hundred guests. There were great snacks and lots of alcoholic beverages. I allowed myself two drinks. I spent more time with Mallory, while Brandy and Carrie floated around the eligible doctors.

One of the doctors was dressed like Santa and eagerly awaited his line of subjects to sit on his lap. I stood in the line as well. Most of the other girls wore suggestive clothing, so his comments somewhat matched what they wore. I still had an enjoyable evening that ended far too quickly.

Working Part Time

I enjoyed the three months I took off to spend time with my baby; but to pay the bills, I needed to get back to work. However, I only wished to work part-time. Ethan was working a day shift, so to avoid paying for

Nursing, Yes I Do!

daycare, I arranged to work the evening shift two days one week and three days the next. I still had to work every other weekend and share holidays as before. I liked the second shift. It was nice not to have to get up at 5:30 a.m. to shower, dress, and get out the door by 6:30 a.m.

At the beginning, I often had to get up many times a night with the baby, but I could just crawl back in bed after I fed him or bring him back to bed with me. The doctors didn't advise against that back then, but still, I sat almost upright with him on my lap and no covers near me.

I missed working with Brandy, Carrie, and Mallory, but most of the girls on the second shift were moms around my age, so we had plenty of things in common to talk about—mostly how we felt we were losing our minds due to lack of sleep and not always knowing if we were doing the right thing for our little darlings. Primary care nursing still worked like a charm on all three shifts.

Working in a local hospital meant I might run into family, friends, or acquaintances as patients in the hospital. For example, my father-in law came to the hospital to have his gallbladder out.

I checked in on him before and after his surgery, and all was well. Suddenly, during my shift, I heard a code blue being called on my father-in-law's unit. Before I could think, the phone was in my hand, and I called the unit.

The charge nurse answered. Before I could say anything beyond identifying myself, she said, "It's not your father-in-law."

I thanked her and went back to work. If that was not enough, later that day, I received a call from the ER with a report on a new patient.

The nurse asked, "Is your husband's name Ethan?"

"Yes, why?"

"A young man down here is named Ethan. He has a back injury and can't move his legs."

My knees wobbled. I plunked into a chair. "What's his date of birth?"

CHAPTER 9 EVENING SHIFTS

It was different from my husband's. I sagged with relief.

The ER nurse said, "Well then, I will give you the report."

When she told me he had fallen out of a hay loft, I said, "Good thing it's not my husband, or I might have wanted to add to his injuries."

The only bad thing about the second shift was getting home at or after 11 p.m. If my shift was hectic at the end, I might not get home until midnight. The first thing I wanted to do was to take a shower before I went near my baby.

Physician as Patient

One warm summer evening, I entered the unit and changed into my scrubs as usual. Then I met with the day nurse for her report. She grinned broadly and pointed to bed nine. "Dr. Nalan was admitted with bacterial meningitis." A sign posted on the door indicated that the room was in isolation, complete with an isolation cart standing outside the door.

Dr. Nalan was a well-respected internist. I was assigned to Dr. Nalan as well as to two other patients with less intense requirements. I checked on my other two patients first and administered their medications, knowing I would be in the isolation room for an extended time.

Isolation is for patients with highly communicable diseases. When entering the room, a person must put on a gown that covers the body from neck to knees, as well as wearing a face mask and gloves. These supplies are all stored in the cart. So, I donned this protective gear before entering room nine.

Inside, Dr. Nalan was wide awake, with a look of discomfort in his eyes. For a moment I felt guilty for not seeing him first, but the day nurse said she had just medicated him.

I greeted him with a caring look. "Dr. Nalan, my name is Aubrey, and I will be your nurse this evening. I'm told you just received your pain medication; is it helping?"

Nursing, Yes I Do!

"No, not yet. I need to be repositioned. Can you do it yourself?" Dr. Nalan was a South African with a heavy accent, but I had no problems understanding him.

"Of course! I'm stronger than I look."

First, I checked his IV. When I did, I noticed it was not working, so I had to pull it out and restart it. When patients have dark brown skin, it can be difficult to see their veins. I usually did well drawing blood or starting IVs on Black patients, but this time I was nervous because he was a doctor. I gathered all my supplies, put on the tourniquet, and—hallelujah—did it right first time, despite sweating profusely.

I then repositioned him, completed my assessment, and gave him his medications. By the time I was ready to leave the room he was sleeping.

Unforgettable Tragedies

During one shift, I was assigned to two patients who had been admitted the previous night after two separate motor vehicle accidents.

The first was a sixteen-year-old boy who had been riding his bike on the road. As a truck passed him, the side-view mirror hit the boy on the back of his head. The boy sustained severe brain damage and was unresponsive to even deep pain. The ventilator maintained his heartbeat and breathing.

The second was a thirty-five-year-old man who had lost control of his motorcycle and had driven through a fence. He suffered multiple bone fractures, lacerations, and severe brain damage. A ventilator maintained his heart and lung operation as well. I spent my first two hours maintaining the ventilators and giving medications, in between speaking with two grieving families.

I kept telling myself, *I have to be strong!*

The doctors were in and out of both patients' rooms.

The sixteen-year-old had so much damage to the vital center in his brainstem that he was not a surgical candidate. Dr. Gold sat down with the parents and spoke with them for approximately an hour about his prognosis.

CHAPTER 9 EVENING SHIFTS

The thirty-five-year-old was brought to surgery to stop the internal bleeding in his brain, but the surgery was unsuccessful. He was also bleeding in his belly. Based on diagnostic tests and his clinical status, Dr. Green told the family we could do nothing to save him. Dr. Gold had already spoken to this family on the day shift about the bleeding in the brain.

Multiple members of the man's family were present. He was a community icon and was a new father to a three-month-old baby. The halls outside the visiting room echoed with cries of sorrow.

Minutes seemed like hours during that shift.

Doctors ordered each patient an EEG to evaluate brain activity. No one was surprised that neither EEG showed brain activity.

I was off the next day. When I returned the following day, I was assigned the same two patients. By this time, both EEGs were flat line for activity. During the day shift, doctors met with each family to discuss removing the patients from life support. Both families signed the consent forms.

The process was to be done on our shift.

Anne gave me the paperwork. "Address the sixteen-year-old first. His parents are waiting in the room with him."

Before I left the desk, the phone rang.

It was the eye bank, asking if the parents still wished to donate their son's eyes. Once a donor has died, there is a narrow window of time during which the eyes can be removed.

I checked with Anne.

"Yes, the consent is already signed. You only need to remove him from life support and call them right after."

I gave the representative that message, and we got off the phone. As I stepped away from the desk, Anne added, "The parents already declined pastoral care."

I nodded.

When I entered the room, introductions were not necessary—they remembered me from two days prior.

"You don't have to say anything," the dad said, his voice thick and hoarse. "Just do it."

I donned my gloves. Turned off the ventilator. Disconnected the ventilator tube from the endotracheal tube. Removed the endotracheal tube from the patient. I gently wiped around his mouth with a gauze.

We all instinctively turned to the heart monitor and gazed at the heart rhythm and rate until it showed a flat line and zero rate. The monitor gave a long beep. I turned it off.

The mother wept, and the dad gave one quiet sob.

I had to speak, though my throat tightened up. "I'll leave you alone but will be right at the desk if you have any questions."

Quickly, I called the eye bank. The parents did not stay long, maybe five minutes. They left the unit quietly.

Within fifteen minutes the people from the eye bank arrived. They thanked me, and while they performed their task, I called the morgue.

The eye bank surgeons left, and the morgue attendants arrived. One of the unit aides came up to me. "Don't worry, we'll do all the postmortem care," she said. "We know you have one more to go."

"Yeah, thanks."

We had all known the schedule ahead of time. The thirty-five-year-old patient's family would not come in until around 8 p.m., which allowed us to take care of the sixteen-year-old in their absence.

Eight o'clock arrived, and I noticed about twenty people in the visiting room. The wife entered the unit with her parents and went right to his room. Slowly, I walked into the room and grasped the wife's hand. She cried and stood closer to me. We just stood there for about five minutes. "Do you wish to have pastoral care?" I asked.

The wife nodded and mouthed, "Yes," though no sound came out.

CHAPTER 9 EVENING SHIFTS

I called the pastoral care office, and in a few minutes Sister Joel entered the unit, She instinctively knew where to go.

After another thirty minutes, Sister Joel came to me at the nurses' station. "They are ready."

I entered the room.

I donned my gloves. Turned off the ventilator. Disconnected the ventilator tube from the endotracheal tube. Removed the endotracheal tube from the patient. I gently wiped around his mouth with a gauze.

This time, the sobbing was much louder. The family embraced one another and Sister Joel.

Fifteen minutes later, the family left the unit. As the door opened, the remaining visitors waiting in the hall began to cry, too. I also heard a couple of screams. Two of the visitors rushed to the wife and embraced her almost too harshly for her little body.

Little by little, over the next twenty minutes, all the visitors for the thirty-five-year-old left. My aides again said they would complete the postmortem care.

"Thanks, ladies. I appreciate it." I left the desk, went into our conference room, and sobbed for ten minutes.

When I returned to the desk, a co-worker said, "Are you all right now?"

I hesitated. "Yes." But it came out as a whisper. I cleared my throat. "Can I help with your patients until the end of the shift?"

She sighed. "Yes, thanks, I have a lot to do."

Long-Term Patients

Approximately eighty percent of patients in the ICU were on a mechanical ventilator, either temporarily or until death. Each night when I arrived home after 11:00 p.m. to my quiet house, I still heard the whirr and hiss of the ventilator and the sound of suctioning sputum from patients' lungs.

At that time, we often performed heroics to save—or prolong—life. Multiple diagnostic procedures and extended respiratory care were often done unnecessarily. At least, that's my opinion, and I am sure others agreed.

A patient admitted with chronic obstructive pulmonary disease (COPD) showing minimal lung capacity would be placed on a ventilator and would have multiple lab tests, X-rays, and more, which appeared to only aggravate the pre-existing condition.

A patient could not be sent home on a ventilator unless the person had twenty-four hours of in-home care, and insurance would not cover it . . . except Medicaid, in some circumstances. They later found out this did not work, either. Patients in these situations were bedbound, with gastric feeding tubes and often a foley catheter. They could not communicate and would develop bed sores despite rigorous schedules of repositioning.

We had one male patient in bed three with COPD whom I'll call Barry. He was on a ventilator and had a catheter in his heart to measure the heart pressure and blood flow, a feeding tube in his stomach, and a foley to drain his bladder.

Barry was obese and, with chronic diarrhea from gastric feedings, he developed a bed sore on his buttocks and a severe rash on his abdomen. We used aluminum paste to treat the abdominal wound and covered it with an abdominal pad—a large dressing for wounds that need a lot of absorbency.

To avoid having to remove the tape every time we changed the dressing, we used Montgomery straps. These are straps with holes for lacings. We placed three straps on either side of his belly, and each strap had two holes to lace shoestrings through. The laces then held the pad in place. We treated the bedsore on his buttocks with a mixture of Betadine, Maalox, and sugar. Believe it or not, this concoction did often help. Barry was in our unit for seven months, during which time we watched him take one step forward and two steps back.

CHAPTER 9 EVENING SHIFTS

We celebrated Barry's seventy-fifth birthday and fiftieth wedding anniversary during his stay. The family brought in cake and champagne to celebrate the anniversary. Anne allowed us each to have a medicine cup of champagne to toast.

In the first four months, we could get him out of bed and put him the chair once during the day shift and once in the evening. It would take three or four of us to do this. We would clamp off his IVs, then disconnect him from the ventilator and pump him with oxygen using an ambu bag during the transfer from bed to chair and vice versa.

For the final three months, Barry was too weak to get out of bed. We saw this by the way his blood oxygen level dropped—he would turn blue around his lips.

Patients on a ventilator cannot eat, so a gastric tube is used for feeding—and the results of this are messy. Calculating the amount and formula for feeding was a challenge because most of the time this caused diarrhea, which only aggravated the skin on their behinds. Barry had diarrhea almost daily.

During the last couple of months, when we turned Barry, he moaned horribly. It broke my heart to see him suffer so.

His doctors did not make time to discuss his prognosis with the family, who would ask the nurses instead. We had no choice but to refer them to the doctors.

The final week of Barry's life arrived before the doctors finally sat down with the family to prepare them for the inevitable. We medicated Barry frequently for the pain all that week. By Sunday, his heartbeat and blood pressure were almost absent. The ventilator continued to push air in, but he had no spontaneous breathing. The family gave their consent to remove him from the ventilator.

They sobbed, but voiced their relief he was no longer suffering. They thanked all the nurses for their devotion to their beloved.

Nursing, Yes I Do!

While we were caring for Barry, we had a similar problem with a female patient in bed four. She also was afflicted with COPD and was on a ventilator, with a feeding tube in her stomach, and foley draining her bladder. Fortunately, she had no bed sores.

She resided in our unit for nine months. She was more alert than Barry and communicated with us frequently, using the magic slate board. Who would have thought such a child's toy would be helpful in the medical profession!

This patient was much easier to get out of bed . . . we could do it with just two people. She had a small family. Even though she was on a ventilator, she would have episodes of being very stable, and we would prepare to transfer her to the medical floor outside our unit. But every time we tried to transfer her, she had a setback, so she stayed in ICU, where we could get her stabilized again. This continued until her death nine months later.

In bed five was a tiny Italian man who had suffered a severe stroke. He was barely responsive—until we noticed a reaction when the women bathed him. Sometimes when day shift was busy, the evening or night shift might bathe a patient who was barely responsive.

Day shift told me about this patient, so I was prepared.

As I started bathing his private parts, I noticed a smile on his face.

I tossed the washcloth on his chest. "Maybe you can wash yourself."

Obviously he could not, but I left the room for a few minutes. I returned with an aide, and we both finished bathing him.

CHAPTER 9 EVENING SHIFTS

The patient in bed six was a ninety-eight-year-old transfer from a nursing home who did not want to be there. Inez was admitted to us after not taking enough food and fluids. She made minimal communication and had a fever of 101 degrees and diarrhea.

As I entered the room with my IV start kit and board, I smiled at the darling little senior and introduced myself. "Good afternoon, I will be your nurse this evening . . . how do you feel?" I laid the IV board on the bedside table.

She just gave me a dirty look.

"Your doctor has ordered an IV in your arm to provide extra fluids. Have you ever had one before?"

Another dirty look.

"May I see your arm?"

She grabbed the IV board from the table and hit me over the head with it. "My doctor also ordered me to come here but never asked me first. I did *not* want to leave the nursing home, and I do *not* want an IV, so leave me alone."

While I was startled by this behavior, I wanted to chuckle. But I kept a straight face and stayed respectful. "I am sorry this has been done against your wishes. I'll contact your doctor immediately. In the meantime, may I get you some ice chips? Your lab tests show you are dehydrated and need some fluids."

She nodded.

"If you can tolerate the ice chips, I am certain we can upgrade to regular fluids."

It was a delightful conversation with the doctor.

"I'm not surprised by her responses," he said, "but the family has made the health decisions for her since her stroke two years ago, and they insisted we do everything to keep her alive."

We agreed to have the family come in and speak with Inez in the presence of the doctor and a witness to discuss her wishes, since she was still of a sound mind.

Nursing, Yes I Do!

The next day the family arrived during my shift.

The doctor stopped at the nurses' station to speak with me before following them into her room. "I had a long phone conversation with the son, telling him what his mother said when she was first admitted to the nursing home six months ago."

Inez had told the doctor she wasn't angry about going into the nursing home, and she was happy with the care. But she knew her body and mind were failing and did not want to be a burden or to suffer before her death. Inez also made sure the doctor knew that she had told all of this to her son, who would not listen. The son thought Inez was too confused to make these decisions.

Inez's neurological status was actually that of an alert person, oriented to her time and place, although she was a little forgetful. Her body was so weak she couldn't maintain a standing position. Having been a dancer in her prime, this was terribly hard for her to accept. Inez understood that this inability to stay on her feet started after her stroke, and her physical abilities gradually declined despite her work in physical therapy.

Once I had gotten this report from the doctor, he and I walked into her room and addressed Inez and her family: her son, two daughters, and their spouses. All of them had tears in their eyes.

Inez and the doctor reviewed her wishes. She gazed at her children. "These are my wishes, and if you love me and do not want me to suffer, you will honor them."

The family members were respectfully silent. The next day, she was transferred back to the nursing home.

In the health care field, invasive procedures like those described above are collectively known as *heroic measures* or *extreme measures* or *life-saving treatments*. I had been working in the ICU almost two years by

CHAPTER 9 EVENING SHIFTS

this time, and this issue of taking extreme measures to prolong the lives of long-term patients with terminal conditions was becoming a real problem for the hospital, the staff, and the family members, as well as the patients. Insurance companies often rejected the costs of these treatments, leaving the hospital to absorb them.

The staff often felt helpless in meeting the needs of these patients, because even so-called *life-saving treatments* cannot reverse the course of a terminal illness, and they usually made the patients feel worse. Family members often felt confused as to why their loved ones did not improve, despite the staff taking extreme measures.

Lastly, the patient often had to endure invasive, painful treatments: multiple needle sticks, suctioning sputum from their lungs—sometimes four times an hour, diarrhea from gastric feedings, muscle, and joint pain from lack of mobility, as well as pain when we repositioned them in bed. Poor blood flow caused skin to break down, which elicited moans and sometimes screams of agony.

Sarah had been attending Quality Assurance Meetings and brought back information to the rest of the staff. She told us the public needed more education on preparing for end of life procedures. This, of course, was not an easy topic to discuss—but needed.

Documents for individuals were being developed in multiple parts of the country. Living wills were just beginning to be used in these types of situations but were still not completely legal. Our state had adopted the types known as Health Care Proxy and Advanced Directive.

A Health Care Proxy document lists an individual who is authorized to make medical decisions if someone becomes incapacitated and unable to make decisions. The Advanced Directive provides specific wishes of an individual, such as *no cardiac compressions* and *no intubation*, for example, if a person's quality of life could not be regained after designated and reasonable attempts of cardiopulmonary resuscitation (CPR).

Do Not Resuscitate (DNR) and Do Not Intubate (DNI) documents were also being used. These required not only the patient's signature, but also an appointed proxy and two witnesses as well as a daily order from the doctor while the patient was in the hospital.

Over the next few months, we saw a decline in the length of stays of the chronically ill patients in the ICU.

Patients who were seen in the emergency room with extreme shortness of breath, a longtime history of COPD, and minimal lung capacity were not initially intubated, as had often been done before. They would be placed on high-pressure oxygen with a mask, and the staff would talk with them, if they were able, and the family would be consulted regarding the prognosis. They were told that the staff could place a breathing tube first down their throat and, if necessary, perform a tracheostomy and place it via the trachea. Oxygen would be needed for the rest of the patient's life, either via an oxygen tank or a ventilator.

Each situation was different, and we did have some cases in which a tracheostomy for long-term oxygen use was appropriate. A speaking valve allowed this type of patient to speak, giving the person a better quality of life.

Chapter 10

BACK TO SCHOOL

I was getting concerned that I might need to go back to school to obtain my four-year degree. My hourly rate was now well above the minimum wage, which was around $5 an hour in 1982. Nurses' wages varied in other parts of the country, ranging from $7.74 to $9.89 per hour for part-time nurses. Of course, the cost of living in any given region has a direct impact on pay, but the income we received did not equal our responsibilities as nurses.

I heard our local Catholic university had a great program for returning students like me. The registration and admission process was quick and easy. All my credits from Christolette College were accepted, leaving me with the need to earn sixty credits.

Working part time and being a mom, I knew I could only handle one or two classes per semester. I started out with chemistry and a required philosophy class. My chemistry professor, Mr. Scott, had salt-and-pepper hair, dark-rimmed glasses, and a dry sense of humor. The classwork was challenging, as was the homework.

The religious philosophy class was mandated by the university. My professor was Sister Cecilia, and she presented a really engaging class, unlike the one I had taken at Christolette. No homework, no exams—just classwork and class participation.

The cost of my classes was $120 per credit hour. This seemed steep, and was a hardship given my income. So, I checked the cost of credit hours

Nursing, Yes I Do!

at the state university, and found they were only $35 per credit hour. I decided to switch to Upstate College of Bastille, also known as UCB.

UCB's campus was about four times larger than the Catholic university, and it had had north and south campuses on opposite sides of the city. The registration and admission process was a bit more confusing, though.

For example, my acceptance letter advised me to go to Saturn B building. So, the day I arrived to register, I entered that building and approached the first worker I saw.

"Oh, they changed the process," she said. "You need to go to Saturn C."

"All right. Do you have a map of the campus?"

"I don't, but it's just out here—she pointed behind me to the front door— "to the left, two buildings down."

Her directions weren't bad. I found Saturn C and proceeded to the registrar's office, where I stood in line for about thirty minutes. There I was given my paperwork to complete. Everyone was patient and kind.

The registrar took my forms and then sent me back to Saturn B. "That's where you'll complete the process to enroll in your chosen classes and provide payment."

So, I hiked back to Saturn B and handed over my paperwork. The clerk there checked my transcript and then looked at me over the rim of her reading classes. "We can't accept the credits from your last chemistry class."

My heart dropped into my stomach. "What? Why?" I did not want to have to repeat a class.

"They didn't include a lab with that class."

"Well, ... can I just take the lab?"

She looked over the transcript again. "Your grade was a 3.3 . . ." She consulted with another person, and they agreed to let me skip the class and just attend the lab. *Whew.*

When I entered the lab for the first time, I was met by Mr. Scott—the professor who had taught my chemistry class at the Catholic university!

CHAPTER 10 BACK TO SCHOOL

I liked chemistry lab, and I guess Mr. Scott did, too, because he was a lot more pleasant in that environment than he had been in my previous class.

My Nursing Therapeutic Communication class was somewhat unsettling. I was unable to complete one of my papers on time because I had a miscarriage. I approached my professor and asked for an extension.

She refused and gave me a zero on the paper. "You'll have to make up the difference with high marks on your other papers."

I already felt hollowed out by my pregnancy loss, but to have the professor react as if I'd slacked off for no reason compounded my grief with frustration.

Therapeutic communication is a combination of conversational skills, including active listening, acceptance, asking questions, and offering encouragement. These techniques are designed to help health care workers better communicate with patients. For this class, we were given a grid showing these various techniques and how to use them.

One assignment was to use the grid as a framework for a report about a situation at work. The instructions said, "Be honest about the outcome even if you could not finish."

I did just that. I indicated that my conversation had to end because a code was called on another patient.

Shock and surprise—my professor gave me a failing grade.

We had to complete another paper with the same instructions. This time, my paper was a fictitious story but followed the grid to a T.

I received an A on that paper.

I never made up another story, and for the rest of the semester, I continued to work hard. My professor saw this, and my final grade was a 3.2. I was okay with that.

In the fall semester before I was expected to graduate, I found out I was having another baby. I had nine credit hours to go and decided to do them all that semester because my due date was May 17, the same day as graduation.

All students were expected to get yearly photos for our IDs. I received a written notice in the mail that told me to go to a building on the south campus for mine.

On the one day I had time to go, the weather was rainy and cold. Traffic was terrible. I finally got to the campus, and as I approached the door, another student was right behind me.

A notice on the door directed us to another building—on the *north* campus. We both gasped and scrambled back to our cars. We pulled into the north campus parking lot at about the same time and scurried to get into the building and out of the cold rain.

Inside, we shook rainwater off our coats and tried not to slip on the wet tile floors as we searched for the right room. As we approached the door where we were to have our photos taken, a young man was locking it.

I said, "We're here to get our school photos."

"Sorry, but I'm closed for the day."

"Listen here!" I cast daggers out of my eyes and used a stern voice I did not think I had. "I am pregnant, cold, wet, and frustrated after being told to go to the wrong location, so I would appreciate it if you would take my friend's picture and mine."

He looked shocked, opened the door, led us into the room, and took our pictures.

My classes for this last semester were Community Health Nursing and an internship in a field of my choice. I chose to do my internship in

CHAPTER 10 BACK TO SCHOOL

discharge planning at St. Christopher's North Hospital. Both experiences were exciting, as they were new to me.

I had always worked in a hospital and often wondered how it would be to work in the community. Our instructor for Community Health Nursing was Ms. Smith, a pleasant, round, gray-haired lady. She had worked twenty years as a community health nurse before going back to school to teach. I was to complete ninety hours over the semester for my internship.

When I arrived at St. Christopher's North, I was directed to the second floor for the discharge planning office. As I entered the room, a very nice, tall, slender, brown-haired girl around my age introduced herself as Tanya. Then, a tall blonde woman about forty years old appeared and introduced herself as Sherrie. Tanya was the discharge planner and worked daily from 7 a.m. to 3 p.m.

Sherrie was Tanya's supervisor and was the director of community services. She frequently attended training related to community services and then shared the information she learned with Tanya, as well as with the therapy department, with whom we worked very closely.

After making small talk and getting to know each other, we discussed my schedule, and the plan was for me to work two days a week for six weeks. This would coordinate with my regular work schedule of three days one week and two days the next. It was only for six weeks, and I could do it. The only thing I resented was having to frequently hire babysitters for my baby boy.

Obviously, on my first day I was a bit nervous while I shadowed Tanya. She made it seem so easy.

"First you need the discharge list." Tanya grabbed a file. "This includes all the patients who will be discharged soon and who might need community services. This is sent to us daily."

She took the file and a clipboard and took me to the therapy department for a meeting. We spoke with the physical, occupational, and speech therapists about each patient's progress. They were a great group of people.

Under Tanya's direction, I used reports from the therapists to make notations next to the names of the patients. Then I read the patient chart for further updates and spoke with the doctors. Finally, Tanya and I met with the patients to discuss their discharge and whatever services or equipment they might need.

North was smaller than the main St. Christopher's facility and was therefore easier to navigate from unit to unit. There was only one unit per floor of medical and surgical patients, and only three floors of patients for discharge planning to see.

On my second day, Tanya handed me my list. "You take the third floor; I will take the fifth floor and meet you on the fourth floor."

Feeling so pleased that I was already trusted to work on my own, I smiled. "Thanks! See you in a bit." I headed to therapy, checked the board for the therapist assignments, and met with the appropriate staff to discuss patient progress.

One physical therapist was assigned to all my third-floor patients, so that made it easy. While he was very knowledgeable about each patient's medical status, he was candid about his opinions on their functional capabilities.

He would say, "After doing my job for twenty years, I can spot a malingerer a mile away."

I headed to the third floor and met with the patient in bed ten—a fifty-year-old male victim of a car accident. He had two fractured ribs, a dislocated right knee, and had possibly had a heart attack, though that had been ruled out. He also had a history of angina, anxiety, and depression. The patient was cleared for discharge by cardiology and orthopedics. Physical therapy recommended a cane because of continued discomfort in his knee.

When I tried to discuss his discharge, he snapped, "I am not ready to go home. I cannot walk, and I had a heart attack, can't you see that?"

CHAPTER 10 BACK TO SCHOOL

I walked closer to him and softly whispered, "We do need to talk about your heart."

His jaw dropped, and I guided him to the chair beside his bed. I sat on the other chair nearby and held his hand. (Touch is one of the elements of therapeutic communication!) I knew the doctor had a lengthy conversation already with him and told him there had been *no* heart attack.

Carefully, I reminded him, "Do you recall the conversation you had with Dr. Cole yesterday about your cardiac test results?"

He nodded.

"Dr. Cole told you there was no heart attack, correct?"

Tears ran down his cheeks. "I need to stay here. I have nothing for me at home."

He held my hands tighter, and I found myself in a fifteen-minute therapeutic conference with him until he was calmer and was dealing better with reality.

When I left the room, I headed back to the nurses' station and informed the head nurse of this. We agreed that we would notify his medical doctor and request a psychiatric evaluation.

My next patient, in bed fourteen, was a forty-one-year-old woman, who had been admitted a week earlier with an exacerbation of multiple sclerosis. She had undergone IV steroids and physical therapy, bringing her back to her baseline of walking with a cane and needing minimal to moderate assistance with household chores.

She was very pleasant and eager to get home to her cat, which was being tended to by her daughter. She had previously gotten a visit from an aide one day a week, as well as her daughter visiting or calling daily.

We set up a van service for her in case her daughter could not take her to medical appointments. I called in the referral to the home care agency to resume her services.

Nursing, Yes I Do!

My next patient was in bed twenty, a seventy-six-year-old female with insulin-dependent diabetes and congestive heart failure. She was independent with her finger sticks for daily blood sugars and her insulin injections. She required oxygen around the clock via a nasal cannula (a tube in the nose).

I sat down with her. "Have there been any changes at home?"

"No, I get around my apartment all right."

"You can complete all your own personal care needs?"

"Yes, no problem."

"What about cooking and cleaning?" The head nurse had already told me the woman's daughter had mental health issues and was not dependable to help at home.

After we had conversed a little longer, she admitted she needed help preparing meals and doing household tasks. We discussed Meals on Wheels and having an aide come in once per week for chores. She agreed, and I put through the referrals.

It was time to meet with Tanya on the fourth floor. "How did it go?"

We chatted briefly, and she looked over my patient notes. We saw patients on the fourth floor, and then it was time for lunch. I was starving, and being with child, I really needed to eat. With this child, I craved cream soup.

After two more days, I was pretty much on my own seeing all the patients on my internship days, and I enjoyed this gig.

Time passed quickly, and before I knew it, my internship was done. Saying farewell to Tanya and Sherrie was difficult. I felt like I left a piece of myself behind with them.

Three weeks before Christmas, I completed my bachelor's program! I assumed I would earn a raise for this, so I asked for an appointment to see Sister Frances in the Director of Nursing office. Later that day, I was called to her office.

CHAPTER 10 BACK TO SCHOOL

"Now that I completed my BSN," I asked, "will I be eligible for a raise?"

Sister Frances put her hand on my shoulder. "Honey, that is all part of continuing education."

My jaw just dropped, and I walked away.

I did end up getting a raise, a whopping twenty-five cents per hour.

Another Maternity

By March 1985, I was feeling fatigued, with the baby due in May. I was not alone, as five other nurses in the ICU were also pregnant. We joked about how long we could keep working before our due dates.

One day I came in and received a report from the day nurse. A priest had been admitted who was very close to the local bishop. "The bishop is expected to come in this evening to visit him."

There I was, a Catholic, but totally naive as to how to greet a bishop. "Am I supposed to kiss his ring?"

"Only if he holds out his hand with the ring facing upward."

I couldn't tell if she was serious. After a couple of hours, the bishop did come in, and I approached him, a little nervously. "My name is Aubrey. Are you here to see Father Ben?"

As I spoke, he raised his hand, but sideways, so I shook his hand with a sense of relief and showed him to Father Ben's room.

My last day was two weeks before my May 17 due date. I had a glow in my face and a bounce in my step. Although I loved my work, it could be grueling, and I felt a relief knowing I would be gone a good, long while.

One of the girls asked, "So how long are you taking off this time?"

I had already decided to take off longer than the recommended six weeks. "Considering I have a three-and-a-half-year-old at home with a newborn on the way," I said, "I entered a return date of 'undetermined.'"

139

Nursing, Yes I Do!

One of the other nurses said, "Don't get too comfortable. You might not want to come back at all."

We all laughed.

After hearing so many positive comments about the Bastille Pediatric Center, I decided to have my second baby there. Fortunately, my doctor had admission privileges there.

I did not want to spend sixteen hours of labor in the hospital again, so I waited at home twelve hours from the onset of irregular labor pains, until regular labor pains were less than a minute long and spaced fifteen minutes apart.

Ethan and I arrived at Bastille Pediatric at 3 p.m. My water did not break despite my ongoing labor pains, so the sac had to be broken manually. The doctor approached me with the longest crochet hook I have ever seen. "This will only hurt for a second," he said.

I held Ethan's hand and squeezed for dear life until the doctor was done. It only took a few seconds but felt like minutes.

Four hours later, I gave birth to a beautiful baby girl who weighed 8 lbs. 3 ounces. We named her Aurora.

I loved being home with my babies, but I was exhausted and began to think work was not as tiring as being a mom with babies. During the nine months I was home, I thought a lot about what I should do as far as work.

I had seven years of hospital work under my belt and was considering home care. My impression was that the level of stress was far lower. I decided to investigate it.

Chapter 11

INTRODUCTION TO HOME CARE

After speaking to a few friends, I learned the United Nursing Care of America or UNCOA was probably the biggest of the home care agencies. I checked them out.

My mom was a great babysitter, so I left my babies with her one morning and drove to the UNCOA Home Care office. I located the human resources department and completed an application to be a community health nurse, commonly known as a CHN. I liked the sound of that.

A week later, I was called in for an interview with a management nurse, Ms. King—a tall, slender woman with long dark hair, who was about my age. She told me she had started as a CHN eight years earlier. "I put in for a management position two years ago," she said, "and I love it. What's not to like! No weekends, no holidays, and no poop." She asked the usual interview questions, including how many hours a week I could work.

"I'd like to work about sixteen to twenty hours a week."

She wrote this down. "You'll have to pass an application exam."

Oh, how I hate tests, but you gotta do what you gotta do.

The test was focused on identifying various medical conditions based on symptoms, along with assessment techniques, pharmaceutical questions, and calculating doses. Fortunately, I passed the test.

Following this, I met with the evening supervisor to continue the interview. Ms. Franklin was short, very round and had wispy, short red hair. She asked me some of the same questions as Ms. King but also questioned me about my knowledge of the city and asked if I had any concerns about going into homes. She was almost scaring me, because I am not familiar with driving around the city, but I convinced her that I could follow a map. I twisted the truth about following a map because I really had little experience doing so.

"You'll have a security guard in your car for all evening shifts," she said. "Do not leave without one."

That gave me some relief.

"We'll issue you a pager," she continued, "and you're responsible to return calls as needed."

This was before cell phones, so we had to use a pay phone or use a patient's phone to return the call.

My salary would be $10 per hour. No health insurance, so I would be on Ethan's plan. I was content with that.

Ms. Franklin closed the folder with my application and her notes. "You'll receive a letter in the next two weeks with our decision."

Two weeks passed. I received the letter—I was given the job. I was scheduled to work evenings from 4 to 8 p.m. various weekdays and every other weekend.

Home Care Orientation

I arrived at my scheduled orientation shift as instructed at 3 p.m. I met with Ms. Franklin, and she introduced me to some of the other nurses, both from the day shift and the evening shift. The girls in the evenings were Cara, Madeline, and Jill. I was assigned to accompany Madeline the first day and Jill the second and third day. They were all around the same age as I was, give or take five years.

CHAPTER 11 INTRODUCTION TO HOME CARE

Before Madeline and I left, we spent a lot of time going over the paperwork and how to write out directions to the house.

I looked over one of the patient files. "Oh, look, those lovely care plans we all hated to do in nursing school are part of the patient's chart."

Madeline chuckled. "Yes, but they're needed. Oh, by the way, home care patients are referred to as *clients*."

Upon making our initial assessment, we identified problems, interventions, and goals. During each visit, we had to address these problems and make changes as needed. We had a specific way to chart our notes, so they were clear to the next nurse.

These clients appeared to be primarily diabetics with wounds requiring dressing changes, people with neuromuscular disorders, those who needed foley catheters changed, and chronically ill people with poor respiratory conditions.

The agency covered seventeen counties, but the unit I was in covered just two. Thank heaven for that.

My Cases

Having someone in the car for these home visits was handy. The men were primarily off duty police officers or security officers, and they knew the area well.

Most of my visits took only fifteen minutes, but if it was a new client, I could be there for one or two hours. First, I took a complete medical history, writing down all the medications, completing a physical assessment, ensuring the person had all his or her prescribed medications and equipment, assessing the home for safety issues, completing treatments as needed, and teaching.

Most of our clients residing in the city were on Medicaid, and one little elderly man angered me a bit one evening. I was to evaluate and dress his wound on his big toe, which had to be done daily. This is a simple task that even a child could do. Moreover, he had enough flexibility to change the dressing himself, but he said he couldn't do it. A nurse was only needed to check the wound's progress twice a week. We were instructed to continue encouraging him to perform his own wound care between our visits.

When I asked if he would consider changing the dressing five times per week and we would come twice a week, he replied, "Why? I pay my insurance to cover this."

I just stared at him. *No, you do not; you are on Medicaid, which comes out of my taxes, and I am also taking care of you.* But I kept my cool.

Granted, people on Medicaid have also paid their taxes, but there is a big difference between using government assistance to provide necessary care and paying a private insurer to provide white-glove pampering.

I felt comfortable with the home visits, and as I entered the lobby of an apartment building for a new case, I quickly ran up the stairs to the second floor.

My guard yelled up at me, "Wait!" He lowered his voice. "That's how the meter reader got it."

I was stunned by his comment. But then I recalled the case, which had recently been in the newspaper. A meter reader was shot upon entering a home to check the meter. I waited on the landing until the guard caught up to me, and he entered the apartment first.

I enjoyed my client load and the care I could provide but hated the extensive paperwork. When I finished my visits, I would drop off the guard in the office parking lot. Then, to make the paperwork a little more tolerable, I would stop at a local doughnut shop to do my charting. Afterward, I'd return to the office and place my charts in the primary nurse's mailbox.

CHAPTER 11 INTRODUCTION TO HOME CARE

On Call

When I first started, only full-timers from day shift took calls from clients in need during the overnight shift. After a couple of months, the agency changed this practice. They asked for a pool of volunteers to cover overnight calls, and the daytime schedule of those volunteers would be adjusted accordingly. I did not volunteer because I was content with my schedule.

One week later, they sent out a memo. Everyone who did *not* volunteer to take calls during the overnight shift would be placed on a rotation schedule, and those who *did* volunteer only had to fill in as needed.

How do you like that!

Because I was a part-timer, my on-call schedule was only two days a month. It was still a pain in the butt. When I go to bed, I prefer to stay there, so I had to recondition myself.

By the way—no security guard accompanied you on night call visits unless you requested a police officer to meet you at your destination.

Disciplinary Action

I thought I was doing a good job. Then I was called to Ms. Franklin's office and told I had not provided sufficient directions to a new client's home. I apologized and said I would improve that. I was given a verbal warning.

One night I was up all-night vomiting. If you had to call in sick, the policy was to call the supervisor directly. By the time I stopped vomiting long enough to make a call, it was 5 a.m. I called in, knowing I would get the answering service.

My hands were still shaking, and I shivered with chills. "I'm not going to be in today," I told them. "If I'm able, I'll call Ms. Franklin during office hours, but in case I can't, I wanted to leave a message."

Nursing, Yes I Do!

The answering service attendant took the message, and I hobbled to bed, exhausted. I was out cold until 9 a.m. and called Ms. Franklin directly. She didn't care that I had called twice. She was upset at getting a message from the answering service.

I was given a written warning.

One night I responded to an overnight call to replace a foley catheter. I arrived at the client's home and, on taking her vitals, found she had a slight fever.

We don't reinsert a foley on a client who has a fever, as we might introduce more bacteria. Standard procedure is to notify the physician, so I called him and gave him a report on the patient's condition. "I don't think this catheter should be replaced, because of the risk of infection."

"Yes, you're right," he said. "Leave the foley out for the night and reassess her in the morning."

All of this was properly documented, and I left a phone message for the primary nurse—a woman I would describe as a bully. She reported me as neglecting my duty to replace a foley. The following morning, she replaced the foley on that client *without* checking with the doctor first.

I was called in again to see Ms. Franklin.

"You've had one verbal and one written warning," she said. "Now I'll have to suspend you."

I was shocked beyond belief. So were my co-workers.

Meanwhile, the doctor followed up and learned that despite his never having received a call with an assessment report, the foley had been replaced. He ordered the nurse to remove the foley and obtain a urine culture.

Since this agency had a union, I wrote everything down and filed a grievance. What a process! I met with the union representative, discussed the issues, and completed the necessary forms. Then I had to meet with the union representative, the director of nursing, and Ms. Franklin.

Ms. Franklin would not admit that she had been harsh or unfair to me.

I told the union representative, "I'm more concerned with having this removed from my record than with getting my job back."

She nodded sympathetically. "We'll see what we can do."

I received a letter lifting the suspension, and all of those disciplinary reports were removed from my record.

Upon going into the office as requested in the letter, I thanked them and stated I would not be coming back. I was very disheartened as I had worked there for less than a year and did enjoy the work.

Back to St. Christopher's Hospital

After much hesitation, I applied at St. Christopher's. After two weeks, I received a call from human resources asking me to come in for an interview.

This time, I met with an alternate assistant director of nursing. Her name was Maggie—what a doll! I liked the fact that she was as short as I was.

"We have an opening for a part-timer on the evening shift in the cardiac care unit," she said.

"Oh, that sounds great! I'm told that unit is a lot quieter, and they tend not to have GI bleeders."

"It's true!" Maggie grinned. Her smile and laugh were truly infectious.

That would be a blessing because that smell is by far the worst. "What's the pay rate?" I asked.

She checked her notes. "It's $12 per hour."

I had heard talk about legislation regarding the poor pay scale for nurses, so the legislation must have gone through.

I am never afraid of learning new tasks, working with new people, or working in a new environment, so I was ready. I met with the head nurse, Ms. Olinkowski. Her hair style was short, wavy, and close to her skull, like you see in movies from the 1940s. She wore dark red lipstick and probably just loose powder face make-up. Her demeanor was direct and firm, and she expected near perfection from her staff. Give this woman a walking stick and she would ram it on the floor for attention. Despite her stern nature, I deeply respected her, as she was extremely dedicated to her patients and the unit.

One thing she said during orientation stood out to me. "Female patients are *not* allowed to wear any lipstick."

I furrowed my brow. "Why?"

She looked at me as if I were the stupidest creature on earth. "How do you look for signs of decreased oxygen in a patient?"

"Umm . . . oh. Bluish color around the lips." The technical term for this symptom is *circumoral cyanosis*.

"Exactly. Lipstick can hide that. So, they mustn't wear it."

The unit had a phase one with seven beds for the more acute patients and a phase two with twelve beds for those less acute, or who were showing progress after being in phase one. The rooms in phase one were all single occupancy, while phase two were doubles. They used primary nursing in phase one but continued with team nursing in phase two.

Initially, I was assigned to phase two. My duties included passing medications, maintaining IVs, and helping the secondary nurse administer treatments as needed.

The secondary nurse for phase two was responsible for vital signs, treatments, repositioning, and hygiene care. This was usually an LPN. We had one aide for phase two who also assisted the secondary nurse.

Usually, three nurses and one aide were assigned to phase one. Sue or Julietta were usually the charge nurse for evenings. Both women were in their early thirties and worked full time. Sue had a face like a china doll and was smart as a whip. Julietta was stunningly attractive with an olive complexion. They were both great to work with, as was the rest of the staff.

CHAPTER 11 INTRODUCTION TO HOME CARE

At times Ethel or Janie would fill in as charge nurses because of the twenty-plus years they had with the hospital. The medical staff included primary physicians and cardiologists, led by Dr. Stone, the chief of medicine. Three of the residents we saw most of the time were Hugh, Christina, and Dan.

Hugh intended to specialize in cardiology. He had quite a sense of humor, was flirtatious, and often approached me singing a familiar song.

Christina and Dan were leaning toward internal medicine. Since this hospital did not perform open-heart surgeries, patients were only treated medically. Patients who needed surgery were transferred to another hospital.

For some reason, I seemed to be slowing down. After a couple of weeks, I found out why. I was with child again—number three. I could not say anything for a while since I had just started working there again.

One cold October day I arrived for my shift. I was hanging up my coat when one of the day shift nurses came into the cloak room to put on hers.

"You won't believe what happened," she said.

I closed my locker. "What?"

"We had a code blue earlier. Sue pulled the code cord and then . . . she just froze."

"Oh. Wow. Then what?"

"Dr. Stone grabbed her shoulders and said, 'Snap out of it!' But she couldn't." She shook her head. "Sue just stood there and cried."

I knew the feeling.

But this was not the first time something like this had happened, so the hospital had to take action. They did what was best and put Sue's intelligence to work in a way that would benefit her and the facility. She was transferred to the cardiac rehabilitation unit, where she could advise, instruct patients, and continue research.

We learned that the position of charge nurse would be filled by Regina, who was a little rough around the edges, so I braced myself in anticipation of her harsh comments.

In addition to dealing with a new charge nurse, I often heard my co-workers complain about working holiday time and late shifts. This was something I did not want to hear yet as I tried very hard to keep my head up and be happy with my job.

Three months had passed, and I would be starting to show my baby bump, so I decided to tell my head nurse and the staff about my pregnancy. They were all very happy for me. Nurses having babies and working close to their due date is not unusual—in fact, it's pretty much routine.

Holiday times were upon us, and the hospital did its usual dinner in the cafeteria, just as it did when I worked the ICU.

Tragedies and Then Some

Our patients in the CCU may have been more mobile than in ICU but were no less critical. Their conditions could change in a matter of seconds.

I recall a patient in bed three—a thirty-eight-year-old man admitted with chest pain, EKG changes, and elevated cardiac enzymes. He had no prior history of heart issues.

I sat with him, took his medical history, and then completed my exam. His last episode of pain had been in the ER about two hours earlier.

I let his wife and brother in to visit and sat at the nurses' station to do my charting. Suddenly, the alarm on his cardiac monitor went off.

His wife ran out of the room yelling for help.

I leaped off the chair and rushed to his room. Multiple staff members from the unit followed. Regina, the charge nurse, escorted the wife and brother to the waiting room.

CHAPTER 11 INTRODUCTION TO HOME CARE

I grabbed the code cart and pulled the STAT—emergency medications routinely used in a code—sodium bicarbonate, epinephrine, lidocaine, a bag of normal saline, and a tray for central line placement.

Another nurse supplied air with an ambu bag until a respiratory therapist arrived with a ventilator. The patient was intubated.

Hugh performed cardiac compressions while the defibrillator was set up. Dan was running the code. He called out for the medications, and I passed them and called them by name as they moved from my hand to his.

The defibrillator was ready and charged. Hugh was closest to the machine, so he delivered the shocks to the patient.

Thirty minutes passed, and the patient showed no response. Although none of us wanted to give up yet, Dan knew it was time. He called the code to cease and declared the time of death.

A mask of misery covered each face as we cleaned up and disconnected the man from the ventilator. All the tubes were left in place in case the family requested an autopsy.

I changed the top sheet to make it look more presentable for the family. I was still in the patient's room with Ethel when we heard the wife's piercing scream and cry.

My heart sank to the floor.

Regina entered, holding on to the wife on the right side while the patient's brother was on the left side. Ethel and I headed out of the room to allow them privacy.

An autopsy was requested, and the coroner took the patient's body out of the room and to his facility. We later found out this patient had a ventricular blowout—the wall of the left ventricle had ruptured.

One of the most unusual tragedies was the time a forty-two-year-old male patient tried to hang himself in the bathroom using a torn piece of a sheet and the shower curtain rod. Fortunately, the roommate heard the noise in the bathroom and yelled for help.

The nurse who ran into the room was August, one of our part-timers from the evening shift, and she stood five feet ten inches. She grabbed the patient by the legs and pushed upward to reduce the pressure on his neck while Janie and I cut the sheet with bandage scissors.

Regina had called the medical staff for an evaluation. They arrived in a couple of minutes. The patient was bruised around the neck and was only semiconscious.

I had not even received a report about him, so I didn't know much. I was later told he had been diagnosed with severe cardiomyopathy (a muscle disease that prevents the heart from pumping blood efficiently). He was advised to retire from his job he loved as an electrician.

After our medical staff evaluated him, they recommended a psychiatric evaluation. When I returned to the room, he was wide awake and very nervous. Dan had ordered Valium to calm him down. We had to talk with him for twenty minutes before he accepted the Valium.

Some emergencies could be a little out of the ordinary, like the time I saw my high school English teacher wheeled into the unit, followed by one of my classmates in a wedding gown.

Yes, she was the bride, and he was the groom. He'd had a cardiac arrest at the altar, and I never found out if it was before or after the "I do."

I spoke with my classmate briefly and comforted her. Fortunately, he did well and was transferred out in forty-eight hours.

CHAPTER 11 INTRODUCTION TO HOME CARE

Oh, yes, there was that successful code called on a darling little eighty-year-old lady. She was admitted with severe atrial fibrillation (irregular heart rhythm) and threw a blood clot that temporarily lodged in a vessel, slowing her heartbeat to a dangerous level, and making her lose consciousness.

After we provided her with all the necessary medications, her heart rate returned to her normal rhythm. As we were cleaning up, I realized I had lost my watch. Janie and I searched all over.

The only place I hadn't looked was the trash. I opened the bin. My gloves! The watch had come off inside the glove that I had pulled off and tossed into the trash bag.

The patient—whom we thought was still unconscious—opened her eyes. "Did you find your watch?"

I chuckled. "Yes, thank you."

It was always exciting to have a celebrity or high-profile patient in the unit. A couple times we had local football players, who did not really fulfill the qualifiers as a cardiac patients but—well, you know—the administration wanted to keep them in a low-traffic area, so they would be placed in phase two. Then we'd try to keep the room free of a roommate or keep the high-profile patient by the window and keep the center curtain closed.

I was being assigned to phase one more frequently and welcomed the work. Ethel and Janie also were happier working with the phase two patients.

Having young guys in phase one during football season was a real challenge. They would hear the televisions carrying the football game in phase two and would insist on being transferred to a room with a television. In some cases, with a doctor's order and agreement of a phase two patient,

Nursing, Yes I Do!

we could wheel the patient to the other patient's room so he could watch the game. It is no secret that stress can aggravate heart function so, in some situations, it was less stress on the patient to meet him halfway. We told the guys, if they started to yell, the TV would be turned off!

Nothing like disciplining adults like children.

At one point, we had a patient who weighed about 450 pounds. We had an extra-large bed, which was large enough to accommodate him. He was intubated and we increased his oxygen percentage from 40 percent to 100 percent; however, that was short lived.

After two days in CCU, his heart gave out. His condition deteriorated regardless of what medications we gave him. We watched his heart rate decline then flatline.

Regina started cardiac compressions.

He was resuscitated for forty-five minutes, but finally the code was called to stop at 9 p.m.

I phoned the morgue and described the patient.

"Oh," the attendant paused. "He's not gonna fit in our drawer."

"What should I do?"

"You'll have to keep him in a cool room until the funeral director can pick him up."

I discussed this with Regina, and we decided to place him in the clean holding room and just lower the temperature in that room. He stayed in that room until the next day when the funeral director arrived.

This man was a recluse with no family or friend to notify of his death.

Chapter 12

MEDICAL ADVANCEMENTS

We heard a rumor of a new drug that would serve as a clot buster for cardiac patients. It was called streptokinase. It had to be given within hours of the onset of chest pain and after confirmation of a heart attack. The drug carried a high risk of the patient hemorrhaging, so a nurse had to stay with any patient given this drug for the first eight hours and take vital signs every five minutes initially, gradually decreasing in frequency. The nurse would need someone to cover her even to go the bathroom.

Our first eligible patient came up to the unit during the night shift before we'd received any training. Fortunately, the medical resident spent most of the time in the room because night shift did not have enough nurses to have one stay in the room constantly.

We had a new nurse who had started working full-time in the unit a couple of months earlier, and who had shown excellent capability with monitoring her cardiac patients and making recommendations to the doctors on medication doses. Her name was Patti, and she took responsibility for the patient during the day shift. She missed her calling to become a doctor.

During the time I was in the CCU, we had four patients on this drug, and only one of those patients was mine. I was initially a bit nervous, but internally I reframed that as *a concern*.

For the first hour, the patient was barely conscious due to the pain medications and eventually became more alert and responsive during my shift.

That wasn't the only high-tech advancement in the CCU. The hospital purchased an intra-aortic balloon pump to be used on patients with severe heart failure. This pump helped the left ventricle of the heart pump more blood out to the rest of the body. It would only be used for several hours or days until the patient would have surgery, such as a valve replacement, or a permanent device implanted into the left ventricle to assist with the pumping.

Here again, Patti took a primary role with these patients, with August and Julietta as her backups. I may not have been as driven as she about the high-tech equipment, but we hit it off well as friends in and out of work.

Life Changes

Ms. Olinkowski had been talking about retiring for a while and finally decided it was time. The hospital scheduled a party at a local restaurant to celebrate her thirty-five years of service.

Her replacement was one of the night nurses, Mrs. Scotnicki. She was average height, slightly overweight, and had curly light brown hair. She spoke with a soft tone in her voice and listened carefully when her staff had concerns. She focused on quality of care and documentation, so our work was constantly reviewed.

Brandy, Carrie, and Mallory, my original buddies from ICU, had all married men making salaries good enough to allow them to stay home and raise their children full-time. We would arrange play dates with the children or an occasional dinner with just the girls.

CHAPTER 12 MEDICAL ADVANCEMENTS

I eagerly awaited my approaching time to go on maternity leave. My new one was due mid-April, so I figured I would work until the first week in April.

This worked out well, because on April 13, I went into labor. My first was sixteen hours, the second was eight hours, and I was thrilled that this one was only four hours.

We welcomed a nine-pound, six-ounce boy and named him Dominick. I had planned to take four months off, and I needed it because he was a colicky baby.

We were blessed with a nice warm spring, and when the baby was ten weeks old, we took all the kids on a trip to the beach. We kept the baby in the shade and hydrated him well. When we came home, I was rinsing out the sandy clothes and toys with the hose while Ethan cleaned the baby.

"Aubrey!" Ethan yelled, "you better get in here!"

I ran inside and saw my baby screaming and turning purple. I grabbed him and checked to see if anything was in his mouth. Then I held him face-down, with his chest in my hand, and patted his back in case he had an obstructed airway. His color returned. "He still needs to be evaluated in the hospital," I said.

Ethan grabbed the car keys. We were about to bundle all the kids into the car, but a guardian angel sent my neighbor to our driveway.

Trembling, cradling the baby against my chest, I squeaked out words. "Please watch Cameron and Aurora for me; we have to rush Dominick to the hospital."

Without hesitation, she directed my two older children to her home.

With St. Christopher's so close by, my mother's instinct would not allow the wait for an ambulance, so Ethan drove to the hospital—running through one red light and pulling into the ER driveway in five minutes.

I ran into the ER and spotted Dr. Brown, one of the residents I knew. "Please take care of my baby! He's not breathing right."

He instantly took him from my arms, and the ER staff rushed to the bedside with the code cart.

Ethan came up and put an arm around me.

I leaned against him. I felt faint, but I took a deep breath to get back to my senses so I could talk to the doctor. I followed the doctor into the treatment room.

Our baby was crying, and his color was a bit pale. They had applied oxygen.

Dr. Brown rubbed Dominic's stomach. "Belly is very firm."

"He is often colicky," I said.

After finishing his initial assessment, Dr. Brown ordered full cardiac, respiratory, and neurological assessments. "I'm concerned about severe reflux," he said, as well as a possible seizure, or . . . some signs of sudden infant death syndrome."

My baby! I trembled, leaning on Ethan, whose posture had gone tense.

Dominick was admitted for two days and discharged with an apnea bradycardia monitor. I do not think I slept deeply for the entire ten months we used this. I was always worried about the wires coiling around his neck, so I would tape them to his back. Despite this, they often came dislodged, and when that alarm went off in the middle of the night, my feet hit the floor before my eyes were open.

He was home only two days when I received a call from my supervisor. "Your four-month maternity leave was not approved. If you don't return this week, you may lose your position in the unit."

My face flushed hotly. "I filled out the form well before I left for maternity leave. Why did you wait so long to tell me?"

She had no answer. I told her what had happened to Dominick.

"Well, if something should happen while you are at work, they would bring the baby here anyway, so you would already be here."

My mouth dropped open. It took me some moments to find words. "I need to be with my baby right now, and if you must take my position away, then do what you have to do."

CHAPTER 12 MEDICAL ADVANCEMENTS

The next day she called me back. "We can hold your position for the four-month leave."

I raised my eyebrows and stifled a grunt. "Thank you."

Starting a New Routine

While I was anxious to get back to work with adults, I hated leaving my three children. After my four months off, I continued to work the evening shift, so my mom and dad would come over about 2 p.m. and stay until Ethan came home about 4 p.m.

I was only back a few days, and the word came down from administration that St. Christopher's was opening a cardiac catheterization lab. This was the first step toward an eventual open-heart unit.

While a coworker and I chatted about this, the code alarm went off, and we rushed out to help.

Sister Serina, a part time supervisor, looked in my direction and said, "Put on your cap."

Not intending to be disrespectful, I replied, "The patient care ranks higher right now."

She gave me a dirty look. I grabbed the code cart, pushed it to the room, and began pulling out the sodium bicarb and epinephrine. As I was doing this, I felt the front of my uniform dampen and realized my breasts were leaking milk. Thank heaven I had a sweater on. It was a successful resuscitation, and I sighed with relief.

Making Changes

After two years on the job, it was 1988 and my salary was up to $14 per hour due to cost-of-living increases and my good performance reviews. But I still felt underpaid compared to the salary for comparable professions.

The CCU was continually understaffed despite being filled with critical patients. I was so tired of the staff gripe sessions, supervisors nagging us to put on our caps, and poor communication between administration and nurses. Finally, hearing from retirees like Ms. Olinkowski that getting the hospital's pension plan was like living on welfare, I decided to rock the boat again.

After putting several ideas down on paper, I went to speak to Maggie, since she was the only one in administration I felt I could trust.

"Listen," I said, "the writing is on the wall. A union might be coming in."

She nodded but didn't say anything.

"I suggest we start a professional nursing committee with four sub-committees: professionalism, education, communication, and recruitment."

She perked up and encouraged me to explain.

The professionalism committee would focus on dress code and work toward eliminating the caps. My research had shown that wearing the cap was originally started by Florence Nightingale and her colleagues to keep their hair out of their eyes and to keep their hair from dropping into wounds. At that time, people then did not bathe as often as we do now, so the cap was cleaner than their hair. Not anymore. The cap is more of a source of infection.

The education committee would focus on properly training the nurses to keep them current in their units or departments.

Communication is vital to keeping everyone on the same page and for maintaining a good relationship between administration and staff.

The recruitment committee would develop an in-house on-call list with incentives for the critical care units. This would help the hospital avoid a potential lawsuit due to poor staffing.

Maggie thought it was a great idea. "I'd love to help you with your presentation."

I was not an avid speaker like she was. "Oh. I had hoped you would present the idea to the staff."

CHAPTER 12 MEDICAL ADVANCEMENTS

"No way' you are!" She turned to the bookcase behind her desk, pulled out a book about oral presentations, and handed it to me. "Read this. It'll help."

As I read the book, I stood and spoke in front of the mirror to practice. It really did help.

Maggie got approval from Sister Frances to hold a general meeting. Each head nurse received invitations to give the staff, and notices were posted in the cafeteria. I had all my reports typed and transferred to clear plastic sheets so I could use an overhead projector.

The day arrived. I was not scheduled to work in the unit that day. We planned a forty-five-minute meeting. I dressed in a suit to look more professional. Maggie was, of course, in her uniform since she worked full time. We sat on the dais with the projector between us. Seventy-seven nurses attended. I was a bit nervous at first, but once I began speaking, the passion took over, and the words flowed. We had signup sheets for staff to volunteer to chair or sit on the subcommittees, and I asked them to call me for details.

It was so exciting to see the interest. Within two weeks we had our subcommittees and scheduled our first meetings. I attended the first meeting of each subcommittee and then let them roll on their own. We set up general meetings every two months. Dates were chosen for the subcommittee meetings and invitations to the staff were posted in each unit, allowing people to attend if they wished.

The next day, as I walked down the hall of the fifth floor, I noticed my memos for five north and five south had been taken from the bulletin boards. I asked one of the nurses about it.

"Someone from the office removed them."

Nursing, Yes I Do!

I checked and they'd been removed from the other floors as well. I was furious and went to Sister Frances's office and asked her secretary about this.

"Sister Frances asked me to remove all the notices."

I found Maggie.

She sighed. "I'll speak to her about it, but . . .I'm going to be handing in my two weeks' notice."

"What? I mean, why?"

"I'm starting a new job in the state attorney general's office."

"Oh. Well, then I'm happy for you." She really deserved that position. "But we'll miss you."

Over the next month, I had to call or visit some of the staff interested in participating in subcommittees, and we held meetings in the cafeteria.

The recruitment committee wanted to hold a wine and cheese party to welcome all the new hires from the past six months. I presented this to Sister Frances, and she agreed.

The plan was to have a friend of mine print out the invitations for free, and I would send them to their homes. The party was to be held at 7 p.m. in the conference room on the second floor.

I arrived an hour early. To my surprise, there was no wine. Instead, the team had substituted iced tea and clear soda. At least we had cheese, crackers, and vegetables.

Twenty-five nurses were on that list, and they all came to the party. A few whispers came my way about the wine and not wanting to upset the new hires, so I said, "We had a last-minute glitch in our plan."

At any rate, the party went well, and I spent time making pleasant conversation with Sister Frances.

The professionalism committee was as determined to rid us of those caps as I was. I developed a letter explaining why nursing caps were no

CHAPTER 12 MEDICAL ADVANCEMENTS

longer appropriate, including my research on the history of caps and how they are a source of infection. I may have twisted Sister Frances's habit, speaking so ill of this long-standing symbol of nursing.

I remembered how excited I was to get my cap when I graduated, but when you get to the workplace, reality kicks in. We were the only hospital in the city—possibly in the state—still wearing nurses' caps.

One of the administration's arguments for keeping the cap was so patients would know who we were. So, I suggested color-coded name badges, possibly with a stripe on them like the stripe on our caps. This was not well received. Four months of convincing passed before it was finally approved to rid the caps.

I had applied for a transfer to the recovery room, thinking the regular day shift and rotation of on call would fit my family schedule better, but it was given to another nurse.

Work in the CCU was getting busier and busier with the more critical patients. I loved working with patients, but again, I worried that I could not safely meet their needs because of the short staffing. I had spent two and a half years in the CCU, and it was time to move on to a job that was staffed better.

I did not even have another job when I handed in my two-weeks' notice. Sister Francis came to CCU the next day and asked why I was leaving.

"I need to be with my children," I said, which wasn't the whole truth.

But she appeared to accept my answer.

Home Care Again?

It was so nice being home again and sleeping normal hours... well, normal for a mom with an eight-year-old, a four-year-old, and a two-year-old.

Nursing, Yes I Do!

One night I fell into bed exhausted because two of the kids had been sick all day. I was out like a light.

But in the middle of the night, Ethan woke me, yelling, "I got it, I got it."

My eyes flew open, and my heart pounded. What was wrong?

His arm came down towards my face. I grabbed his arm. "No, you do not got it."

He was still asleep. Probably dreaming he was playing baseball.

I had an adrenaline rush that kept me awake awhile longer, but he hadn't awakened the entire time.

Looking through the want ads never really appealed to me, but after a few weeks, I knew I needed to get back to work. It was difficult to budget one salary for five people. Working in another hospital was not an option; staffing problems would be the same.

An acquaintance told me about an opening with the company she worked for, Total Care. They needed a nurse to put together policies and procedures and to provide in-service training for the medical staff as needed. That sounded wonderful.

The interview was scheduled, and I dressed in dress pants, blouse, and jacket. When I arrived, the receptionist wrote my name and the reason I was there.

She then looked me up and down. "Slacks are not allowed in this office."

I apologized and sat down. In a few minutes I was called for my interview into a fabulous office and met with the owner, his wife, and the office manager. The owner described their home care business, clients, and the area they covered. I was told they took their clients on a yearly boat trip. By this time, I realized this company catered only to the wealthy.

CHAPTER 12 MEDICAL ADVANCEMENTS

Their initial questions were basic, but then the manager asked, "So do you plan on having more children?"

I had to stop my jaw from dropping, as it is inappropriate and unethical to ask that. I blurted out the first response that came to mind. "Why?"

"We need to ensure your employment isn't interrupted by childbearing."

Eeeks! Politely, I replied, "I cannot guarantee I will not have more children and wouldn't want that to cause a problem for you, so I may not be the right person for you."

The owner asked if I knew of someone else. "We prefer to interview people recommended by someone we trust."

I took that as a compliment. "Thank you. I may have, but I'll need to check with her first." I had in mind someone I knew was not planning to have any more children because of her age.

When I left, after a few sighs on the ride home and telling the story to my husband, I called Callie.

She was receptive and said she would call.

I called their office to give them her name and said she would be calling. It worked out well for Callie and for me as well, because once she was working there, Callie asked if I would mind picking up some private duty cases. "They may only pay LPN rates," she said, "but they're low stress."

I agreed.

My cases were primarily in clients' homes. Occasionally I would have a patient in the hospital, and the family would privately pay for a nurse to supplement the hospital care. The home care cases were primarily bed-bound patients being cared for by a family member who needed respite. I gave a lot of bed baths, tracheostomy care for patients with home ventilators, and lifted people out of bed with a mechanical lift. One client was a young girl with muscular dystrophy, and I transported her from her room to the other side of the house so she could sit in a recliner and gaze out their picture window.

Nursing, Yes I Do!

One of my hospital patients was Mr. G, a sixty-year-old well-respected businessman who had suffered a massive stroke. Because he was generally a strong man, he showed great progress. I earned much respect from his family, and they joked about taking me home with them. Those kinds of comments keep me in this profession.

Working with the hospital patients, we had to be careful not to step on the staff's toes. I was responsible for providing all personal care, medications, and treatments, so I had access to the chart, medication, and treatment book. If I needed to give a narcotic, I had to ask the staff nurse to supply me the medication from the narcotic cabinet—I did not have access to the keys to the cabinet. This work was more relaxing, and despite having three small children at home, I was not stressed out.

After two years, Callie was ready to leave due to frustration with upper management and their demands. When she told me, I decided to wait and see how the chips would fall.

Sure enough, management asked if I would consider the management position Callie had just left—the same one I had turned down because I couldn't guarantee I would not have any more children.

I really liked this work, but the business was slowing down, so I said, "It's not right for me, but I hope you find someone."

Besides, our family needed more money than I was making doing this kind of home care, so I looked elsewhere again.

Chapter 13

SUPPLEMENTAL CARE

Well, back to the want ads. An agency called Supplemental Care had an opening for a part-time home care nurse on an infusion team.

I made an appointment with Franchesca, better known as Frankie. I arrived at a warehouse-type building in the inner city. There was no receptionist, so I walked around until I found Frankie in a back office. A man with her identified himself as Neil. Frankie was a slender, blonde, blue-eyed woman in about her late twenties. Neil was a dark-haired, dark-eyed, well-built man about the same age.

They asked me to sit down and began rifling off questions. They had so many questions, but for some reason, I felt comfortable with them. These people were real—no fake presentations. They weren't the owners of the company.

"The company has two departments," Frankie said, "medical equipment, and an infusion team. The infusion team is—" he waggled his finger between himself and Frankie. "But we're adding one person and, if business increases, another."

Apparently the interview went well, because Frankie called me the next day to give me the job. "We'll need you to return with a copy of a physical completed within the last year."

I quickly called my primary physician to schedule an employment physical for the following week.

Nursing, Yes I Do!

In the meantime, Total Care ceased operations—for reasons that were never disclosed to me—so I didn't have to resign.

I met with Frankie and Neil to go over the paperwork. During this visit, I asked more questions about them. They had each worked in hospitals for about five years and then home care in another agency for the previous four years.

Neil said, "This agency was previously managed by someone else—"

"Oh, who?" I asked.

He waved away my question with one hand. "It's not important. They were unable to continue."

"Right now, the staff is just the three of us," Frankie said. "We have a client load of only ten, so we can handle it.

It was decided I would work per diem and get paid $20 per visit, as well as receive reimbursement for mileage.

Starting an IV on a patient varies in levels of difficulty. I followed the same general practice as my colleagues, calling each patient a day before my appointment to advise them not to smoke or drink coffee, but to drink as much water as possible on the morning of our visit. This makes the veins easier to see.

I generally sought to use the cephalic, basilic, or antecubital vein in the mid to lower arm. The cephalic vein is on the same side as the thumb, the basilic vein is on the same side as the pinky, and the cubital vein is in the middle. If, upon my arrival, the veins remained difficult to see, I applied a warm soak for a few minutes. Most often, this did the trick.

But some patients are just harder to stick than others. One patient, a stout middle-aged woman, had small, slippery veins. I tried the antecubital vein and got nothing. "Sorry. Let me try a different vein."

The basilic vein also evaded my needle. "Oh no," I said, I'm so sorry."

I tried a smaller needle, one meant for children. But when I tried the cubital vein, it also slithered out of the way. "I can't stick you again," I said, my cheeks flushing. "I'm going to call my supervisor."

CHAPTER 13 SUPPLEMENTAL CARE

"Don't worry about it," the patient said. "Happens all the time."

I called Frankie and explained. "I could not access a vein after three attempts." She sighed. "Okay, I'll come over and do it."

This was a rare occurrence, but it was terribly embarrassing for me, so I resolved to improve my skills.

For the first three months, I completed about five to ten visits per week. Most of my visits were to chemotherapy clients who required a neupogen injection to boost their white blood cell counts, intravenous infusion for hydration, and education on their medical conditions, medications, and diet. My patients varied in levels of illnesses and resided in rural, urban, and suburban areas. Most of my visits were completed in half an hour, so the money was good. I really enjoyed this.

One of my patients had a pet bird that looked like a macaw. I had never seen such a large bird—and one that talked! When I arrived at their home, I heard a voice making the sound you hear at a hockey game when a score is made. He also made the sound of a ringing phone and then followed by saying, "Hello." It was a nice distraction and provided a topic to speak about with my patient while I was starting an IV and administering a steroid infusion over the next two hours.

The client log was growing, so Frankie hired another nurse. Her name was Connie, and she had previously worked with Neil. Connie was tall, had short blond hair, and was well endowed. She was not as down-to-earth as Frankie and Neil and could be somewhat full of herself. At any rate, we all worked together well.

169

We began to receive referrals for multiple sclerosis clients who needed intravenous steroids once a month and possibly a change of their foley catheters. I knew this was coming—on-call rotation; ugh.

Both Connie and I had small children, so Frankie and Neil took the on-call duties most of the time. Connie and I took calls only if the other two were unavailable, which was rare.

Frankie wanted to relocate our office, and she found a cute little place just south of downtown and across the street from Park Place, the pharmacy where we picked up our injectable medications. This location was only a seven-minute drive from my home, as opposed to the twenty-five-minute drive to the other location.

The Buyout

Rumor had it that Total Care was venturing into home care again. I am not quite sure what the process was, but after seeing our success, they invested in the company. Shortly thereafter, Total Care bought Supplemental Care entirely.

The manager at Total Care demanded that we reopen all our Supplemental Care cases under their name. During this time, we felt an uncaring attitude toward us, and we took a cut in our pay.

Total Care did not have a great reputation, and the physicians who were our primary clients were dissatisfied with them and stopped sending us patients.

Frankie, Neil, Connie, and I had a meeting with the Park Place Pharmacy staff, and we were all impressed with them. Park Place agreed to inquire about purchasing the infusion team from Total Care. I began to feel like a piece of meat for sale.

Frankie worked her magic and spoke to the physicians who were dissatisfied with Total Care, asking them if they would reconsider using us if the infusion team were a separate entity owned by Park Place. She knew

CHAPTER 13 SUPPLEMENTAL CARE

the physicians had worked with Park Place for many years, so she didn't think it would be a problem—and she was right.

Park Place offered to buy just the infusion team from Total Care, and there was a verbal agreement, but before the paperwork was signed, the owners of Total Care refused to sell because our team again had an increase in business.

Frankie informed two of our biggest providers that our infusion team would be working for Park Place in the near future, so they discharged their clients from Total Care and admitted them to Park Place. Neil, Connie, and I had not signed noncompete agreements, although Frankie had, so the three of us could see Total Care clients for Park Place once they were transferred.

The charts for the few clients who were still admitted to Total Care were placed in a locked cabinet by the Total Care staff. This was beginning to look like a messy divorce marriage. Fortunately, after a couple of weeks, Total Care signed our team over to Park Place Pharmacy.

Things went well for about six months, and I regularly made ten visits per week. If I had a two-hour infusion, that counted as two visits.

They say all good things come to an end, and after a year Park Place Pharmacy was no longer able to pay us, so we again sought a good home.

Frankie pounded the pavement and found an agency that needed an IV team. Their name was HCS, and they had both a licensed and a certified side. Briefly, the licensed division provided short-term home care services through specific private insurances, as well as short- to long-term services paid by patients out of pocket. A certified home care agency provides short-term home care services covered by Medicare, Medicaid, or private insurance. Our team would be on the certified side, and we would be paid a salary rather than an amount per visit.

When the four of us started, we had enough work to keep us busy without being overwhelmed. Since this was a large, for-profit business, they depended on us to bring in more business, and we did. Within three months, we doubled our client load and hired two more nurses.

At this time, Frankie needed a title, so she was appointed assistant director of patient services or ADOPS . . . a funny-sounding title so we could tease her.

The person hired as the director of patient services was Meredith Hallorey, someone from my past life. She had been the head nurse in the ER at BCH. Meredith and Frankie hit it off great. We needed another nurse as well, so we hired a male nurse named Glen.

The business grew, meaning I often left my youngest, who was still not in school, with sitters. Then I received an opportunity to work weekends. As bad as it sounds, it worked out great. I worked three hours on Friday afternoon to get my assignments and answer calls with referrals. Then I made visits on Saturday, Sunday, and Monday, and was responsible for any additional visits up to 5 p.m. After that, the full-timers were on call. If I had a wedding or something else going on during a weekend, I only had to ask one of the team to cover me, and that was rare.

It was nice being on salary; however, after I did the math, I learned I was making $14 per hour. I didn't complain, though, because my scheduled visits were usually done by 2 p.m. or 3 p.m., and I only had to be on call until 5 p.m.

Those Strange Calls

I learned to be on guard and protect myself while going into homes. I carried pepper spray and had an alarm on my key ring that was intense, ear piercing, and could be heard for approximately a quarter mile.

One Saturday morning, I left to visit my four clients on a route that would cover about one hundred miles round trip. I started with Alan,

CHAPTER 13 SUPPLEMENTAL CARE

a diabetic patient living in a rooming house. I was covering this client for the licensed division, which we did at times. I was to review teaching him how to perform a finger stick to check blood sugar and was to instruct him about his diet and medications.

I arrived at the big farmhouse-style residence, walked up the porch steps, and rang the doorbell. No answer. I knocked. Still, no one answered the door.

I checked the client's record—he had no phone number listed, or any family or friend contacts. I knocked again and waited about ten minutes. I decided to see my next client, fortunately just a few minutes away, to do a follow-up assessment on her cancer treatment and give a neupogen injection.

Once that was done I returned to Alan's rooming house. Again, no answer.

My third client was twenty minutes away, and there I was to administer a two-hour steroid infusion that needed to be done at the scheduled time.

This was during the early 1990s, before most of us had cell phones. So, I drove until I found a phone booth. I called the police because, for all I knew, Alan could be keeled over on the floor.

When the dispatcher answered, I explained the situation. "I need to check the patient's medical status and ensure he took his medications." If the client's health or safety was in jeopardy, I trusted the police to take the necessary steps to send him to the hospital.

"I understand ma'am," the dispatcher said. "Do you have a number where the responding officer can reach you to follow up?"

I gave the dispatcher my pager number. "The officer can page me when they find him, and I'll call them back."

Next I called Neil, in his role as supervisor, to keep him updated.

I went to the home of client three, Emily, and got her situated in her bedroom with her infusion. An hour had passed, and I had still received no page from the police department. "Do you have a phone I can use?"

"Yes, you can use the one in the den." She directed me down the hall.

Fortunately, the den was out of earshot from Emily's bedroom, so I could maintain Alan's patient privacy. I called the police department to follow up on him.

Finally, my call was transferred to the right officer. "Yes, ma'am, we were able to enter the apartment. The man was sitting at his kitchen table and appeared fine to us."

I thanked him without asking why they hadn't paged me.

Once Emily's infusion was complete, I had a twenty-minute drive back to Alan's home. I got out of my car and held my breath for a minute as I walked up the porch steps.

This time when I knocked, an unkempt, middle-aged woman answered the door.

"I'm looking for Alan," I said.

She pointed up the stairs to a large middle-aged man standing on the landing, wearing nothing but a towel wrapped around his waist.

Another man's head poked out of a doorway behind Alan. He waved. "Hello."

I gasped and said to the Alan, "I am your home care nurse assigned to see you today . . . I will wait until you get dressed."

He replied, "I am dressed."

I had my pepper spray and alarm available. I followed my gut feeling that I was safe and went upstairs to complete my visit. At least the second man was fully dressed, and he welcomed me into the apartment with a pleasant demeanor.

We stood awkwardly around the kitchen table. There were no chairs. I have no idea where they had gone.

Alan was very quiet. His client record showed that he had a learning disability.

CHAPTER 13 SUPPLEMENTAL CARE

"I'm here to review your regimen. Do you have your glucometer?" This device checks a person's blood sugar with a needle stick on the finger and records the levels.

He looked at me blankly, while the other man rooted around in a drawer.

"Did you eat?" I asked Alan.

"Yes."

"And did you check your blood sugar?"

"Umm . . . no."

I checked the time. It was 1 p.m.—five hours later than his original appointment. I was starting to worry about how that might affect his health. "Did you take your insulin?"

"Yes, I did that."

"Okay, good. Let's check your blood sugar."

Alan's friend had found the glucometer and brought it to me. By this time, I was so nervous my hands were shaking, and I accidentally broke the glucometer. "This is not working. Your doctor will want to check your blood sugar. I can draw one from your arm; is that all right with you?"

"Yes."

Since there was no chair for him to sit down, I drew the sample with him standing. Thankfully, I had no problems getting the blood sample.

I packed up my things. "Please make sure someone is available to answer the door for the regular nurse when she comes tomorrow."

Alan nodded. "Yes, I will."

"I'll arrange for the medical equipment company to deliver you a new glucometer."

"Thanks."

Alan's fully dressed friend showed me to the door.

I saw my fourth patient—an uneventful visit, thankfully—and headed for the hospital to drop off Alan's blood sample. As I drove, I realized I

Nursing, Yes I Do!

needed an order from the doctor for the blood sugar test. I pulled up to another phone booth to call the doctor.

I explained everything that had happened, including calling the police and finding Alan wearing only a towel. The doctor chuckled.

"He did eat and took his insulin," I said. "When I tried to take a random blood sugar, the glucometer didn't work"—my cheeks flushed all over again— "so I obtained a venous sample, assuming you would want that. But I need an order. May I have one?"

"Yes, of course."

I went to BCH to drop off the sample, called the equipment company, and went home, glad that day was over.

I was working Memorial Day weekend, and one of my cases was a new admission for IV antibiotics. As I drove down the street, I noted his home was in a poor and run-down neighborhood. I parked the car and unloaded my supplies—my nursing bag, a tote of IV supplies, and an IV pole.

As I walked across the street, a young gentleman approached me. "Whatcha got in the box? Is it lingerie? Are you the lingerie lady?"

I just smiled. "No, they're work supplies."

Thankfully, he walked away before I got to the other side of the street.

My client was Ricky, a quiet, middle-aged man diagnosed with chronic cellulitis of the leg. This is a bacterial infection that causes a rash, swelling, and pain, among other symptoms, and can be life threatening.

I completed my assessment and gave him some instructions on how to care for his cellulitis. We also discussed his diet and medications.

I started the IV in his left forearm and placed the top of a new tube sock over the IV site to keep it clean and gave him an extra one. I used to buy packs of them at a discount store and just cut off the feet. They worked great, and patients could wash and reuse them.

CHAPTER 13 SUPPLEMENTAL CARE

I administered the first dose, and Ricky had no reaction. "You're supposed to get a dose every six hours, so I'll teach you how to administer these yourself."

He looked wary. "Seems complicated."

"The steps are actually really simple."

I taught him the SASH method: saline, antibiotic, saline, and heparin. Saline is used to flush the IV before each dose of antibiotic. Then, after the antibiotic was done, the IV was flushed again with saline and then a weak heparin solution. He did well.

I started packing my tote. "Since I was here for your noon dose, I'll return at 6 p.m., and hopefully you'll be able to administer your midnight and 6 a.m. dose. Then I'll be back tomorrow at noon to check the line."

"Nah, I got it. You don't need to come back at six."

"All right but let me at least call you and walk you through it."

"Sure, that sounds good."

I had not been taking client calls after 5 p.m., but I had been asked to fill in over the holiday weekend, and I would be paid an on-call supplement for an after-hours call.

So, we talked at six, and he did well administering his dose, based on his responses on the phone.

That night I was jarred from sleep by the ringing phone at 11 p.m. I jumped out of bed to answer it. The on-call coordinator told me to call Ricky.

When I called him back, Ricky said, "My IV came out, so I won't be able to give myself the medicine."

"I'll be right there." I tossed on jeans and a sweatshirt and drove to his home.

When I arrived, many people were visiting.

Ricky confessed, "I couldn't enjoy the party with this thing in, so I pulled it out."

I gave him my best "mom glare." "Do you realize how important this medication is to heal your cellulitis?"

He ducked his head and nodded. I restarted his IV and administered his midnight antibiotic dose—that took more than thirty minutes.

I went home and crashed.

The next morning, I relayed all this to Glen.

He said, "I'll see him at noon and give him a piece of my mind."

Yippee, one less visit for today!

Then there was that wonderful gentleman who would not get out of bed and lay there under a sheet, naked. After what happened with Alan and his towel, I was learning to be even more on guard.

When I arrived at this man's home, his mother, a frail, feeble woman, let me in and directed me upstairs. As I approached him, he looked me up and down.

I kept my distance as much as possible, getting close only to take his finger stick blood sugar, blood pressure, pulse, and respirations.

This time, I was reporting to Neil, who winced at the story. "I'll take that patient tomorrow."

The next day Neil returned from that call and said that when he arrived, the man was lying there naked with semen all over the front of him. "He thought you would be returning."

"Ugh!" Was I ever glad Neil had taken that call.

Going out to the rural areas was always interesting. I should have known better than to wear white slacks.

I had an appointment to administer a two-hour methylprednisolone infusion to a patient who lived on an old farmstead. As I approached

CHAPTER 13 SUPPLEMENTAL CARE

the door, I saw an animal the size of a baby bear. His head was twice the size of mine; his bark hurt my ears. I am not afraid of dogs, but this one was very big.

Inside the house, I heard a female voice. "Bear, leave the nurse alone." My client came to the door and smiled.

"Hi, I'm Aubrey. I'm here for your infusion."

She let me in, and Bear stared at me while I inserted the needle in his owner's arm. Thank God, it went in the first time.

I sat down to do some charting and patient instruction. Within a couple of minutes, Bear dropped his head on my lap. My white slacks were not white after that.

"He obviously likes you," the client said. "You can pet him."

I scratched behind his ears, and he apparently was a big baby, loving every minute of it.

Navigating the Native American reservation was a real challenge. Remember, this is before GPS. Cell phones existed, but few people had them. Home care nurses still used pagers for communication. Then you had to find a phone booth or ask to use your client's phone.

I had two clients to see on a reservation, and I decided to make that my first stop that day. My map was in the car, and I had already looked at where I had to go before I left the house. I had some directions from the hospital discharge planner, because the first client was a new admission, and she had no phone.

I was to drive forty miles down Route 7A, turn right at Tom's Smoke Shop, drive two more miles, turn left at the corner with the mobile home with the red tire on the lawn, drive 1.7 miles and pull in the drive path at the green and white mobile home with the German shepherd out front. I found it . . . great!

I knocked on the door and was greeted by a young boy of about twelve. I introduced myself. "I'm here to see Mrs. A."

He led me to a back room where a very elderly Native American lady sat in a rocking chair.

I introduced myself. "How do you feel?"

She whispered, "Fine."

I explained why I was there. "Do you have any questions?"

She shook her head.

Her medical conditions were chronic obstructive pulmonary disease and chronic renal failure. I took her temperature, pulse, respirations, and blood pressure, as well as a complete body system assessment. All the readings were within normal limits. She was independent in navigating within her home, and her family assisted with her personal care, drove her to appointments, and paid her bills.

When I asked where her medications were, she pointed to a drawer next to her. There were five bottles of pills, all up to date. I wrote down the names, doses, and frequencies. I held up each bottle of pills and asked Mrs. A if she knew what they were for. She was able to explain the purpose of three of the five. I advised her about the other two.

"Do you have any questions about your medical conditions?"

"No."

I reviewed her diet with her and gave her some meal plan suggestions. "What kind of exercise are you getting?"

"I walk two miles every day."

"Excellent! That's everything for today." I said good-bye.

My next client was down the road behind the smoke shop. He was also a Native American. He was a bilateral amputee after having been in a horrific car accident two years earlier. He was not new to the agency but had just gone through a setback, having had a mini stroke.

CHAPTER 13 SUPPLEMENTAL CARE

I had some of his old assessments so I could compare, but I asked him if he felt any different.

"I only feel weaker in my right hand."

My assessment found his vital signs normal, his heart and lungs sounded normal, his visible skin was intact, and he denied any skin breakdown elsewhere. His right-hand grasp was weak, but he capably maneuvered his manual wheelchair.

He was not on any medications because he refused to take any more pills; he had left the hospital two days earlier. Functionally, he was independent with all of his personal care, meal prep, and getting into and out of his wheelchair.

"What about other exercise?" I asked.

"I go to the gym and work out with a trainer three times a week."

"Are you able to do your errands and get to appointments?"

"Yeah, I have a friend who drives me."

"All right, that's great. I don't see any further issues that would require us to keep your case open, but do you feel you need further nursing visits or home therapy?"

He replied, "No."

"Okay. I will tell your doctor about the issue with your right hand."

He nodded and showed me out. Working with patients on the reservation helped me develop a better understanding of the Native American culture—not only their sense of pride, but how they care for one another.

Patient from the Past

One day Ethan called me to the phone at home. "It's a Mrs. G. Says you treated her husband when you were with Total Care."

I took the phone, racking my brain. "Hello?"

"Aubrey, I'm so glad I found you! My husband had another stroke."

Nursing, Yes I Do!

As she described her husband's condition, it came back to me. This was the family who had wanted to take me home with them.

Mr. G was back in the hospital and had been given a short time to live. "I called Total Care," Mrs. G said, "and they don't have staff nurses to fill hospital shifts anymore, so I thought of you. Do you know enough nurses to fill all three shifts, or could we do twelve-hour shifts in the hospital and then at home? We can pay $25 an hour."

How could I say no? I could schedule this around my part-time day cases. "Yes, I can get a couple of more nurses to do this for you."

My first call was to Iris, who had worked on Mr. G's case with me at the agency. "Yes, I can do days," she said.

We decided twelve-hour shifts would be best. I asked her to recruit a couple of more nurses, as she currently worked three twelve-hour shifts in the ICU at the hospital.

I then called Glen. "Would your wife be interested?" She was an RN and was extending her maternity leave from the hospital. "I thought she might be interested in some low-stress work."

She said yes as well.

I could do two twelve-hour night shifts per week. I called Mrs. G back, and she was relieved. "Mr. G will be discharged in two days. Can you meet us at the hospital tomorrow to discuss the plans? Then we can start when he gets home."

"Yes, that sounds perfect."

Mr. and Mrs. G lived in a beautiful mansion of a home, complete with housekeepers and a butler. Working the night shift, I did not have any encounters with the staff.

I found it a little strange to be in that beautiful old mansion while everyone slept. I would bring books and needlepoint to keep me busy between medical tasks.

CHAPTER 13 SUPPLEMENTAL CARE

Within a short time, we knew Mr. G's time would be up soon, as he gradually became weaker and weaker. I recall an episode when I needed to boost him up in bed so he could breathe better, and I had no helpers. I positioned myself at the head of the bed with my knees just behind his head, wrapped my arms under his armpits and brought him upwards pretty much onto my lap. At this point, he was only semiconscious, so I was not concerned about my body position.

This case fit around my home care visits, and I continued there for about six months until Mr. G died. For years afterward, his wife and I sent each other Christmas cards.

One year, the cards stopped. I assumed she joined her husband.

Rethinking Home Care

Things went smoothly at HCS Care for about two years, except for Connie leaving. She took a job in a doctor's office, administering intravenous chemotherapy.

By 1994, we had four full-timers plus me covering the weekends. Neil continued to be our supervisor, and Frankie was promoted to director of patient services after Meredith took extended time off.

After a while, problems arose in the upper management of the company, and eventually, Frankie and Neil had enough of it. When Frankie found out she was pregnant, she handed in her notice rather than taking maternity leave. Neal took a supervisor job at another company. I decided to stay where I was, but soon realized this was a mistake.

Daria was the new director of patient services, and she struck me as unstable.

I came in one Friday and noticed she had her six-month-old baby boy sleeping in a box in her office. I heard him cry while she was on the phone, so I picked him up to soothe him. I calmed him down. When she got off the phone, I said, "If you need me to, I can keep him in my office until 5 o'clock."

"Yes, thanks."

While I had the baby in my office, I overheard her conversations with other staff members and the sound of her office door slamming twice. At five I took her baby to her.

She was obviously distracted, as she never even made eye contact with me. I laid the baby down in the box. Fortunately, he did not cry.

I said "bye," got no response, and quickly headed out the door.

I had recently had an evaluation that praised me for being a valued member of the company with a grade of ninety-eight percent.

We were losing intravenous cases on our certified side, and I was seeing more and more traditional cases from the licensed side. I didn't mind this, but too many new cases from the hospital were being sent home with no plans in place.

I was the one calling oxygen supply companies for oxygen in the home, durable medical equipment companies for walkers, wheelchairs, shower chairs, etc., and pharmacies for medications.

I was working one holiday when I was sent to see a gentleman who'd been sent home from the hospital without oxygen or medications. I looked over his chart, hardly believing he'd been released. "All of that should have been set up by the social worker at the hospital. Did they tell you anything?"

"No, they just gave me some papers to sign and sent me home."

"Do you have family nearby? Or friends who can help?"

He shook his head. "Just you all."

He was scheduled to have an aide just a couple of hours per day. Other than that, he was in his apartment, alone.

I tried to call the oxygen supply company and the pharmacy, but they had closed early for the holiday. It was not a safe discharge, so back he went to the hospital.

CHAPTER 13 SUPPLEMENTAL CARE

This kind of thing was happening far too much.

Back at the office, I made my complaint to Daria.

"Well, the hospital complained that you sent their patient back," she snapped.

"Seriously, what did they expect me to do? It was an unsafe discharge!"

She did not care.

I later found out that Daria took my evaluation, removed my name, used it as a template for another worker, and proceeded to cut my hours.

I saw the writing on the wall and handed in my notice.

Chapter 14

WORKING THREE JOBS

In 1995, we moved to a larger home in a new school district, so I decided to apply to be a substitute school nurse with the local school district. I was called in for an interview and met with the assistant superintendent. I was asked if I would fill in for some classes as well, and I agreed to teach science-related classes.

Then I received a call from Neil. The company he worked for, Chapel Care, needed more nurses with intravenous experience, and I could work part-time.

I *also* received a call from another co-worker in home care, seeking a home care nurse for occasional IV cases, as well as filling in a night shift here and there. He had also briefly worked for HCS Care. This agency was called Regency Home Care.

My favorite option was working in the school district, so I gave Neil availability for two days a week and the other home care job one day a week.

Regarding the school job, I was told I would be called by about 5:30 in the morning if they needed me, so I told them which days of the week I would be available. For some reason, when that phone rang at 5:30 a.m., I woke up in a snap and answered the phone as if I had been awake

CHAPTER 14 WORKING THREE JOBS

for hours. The staff member who would call me was a very pleasant young lady, so it was not hard to return the pleasantries.

The first couple of times I was called, I was assigned to work alongside the full-time school nurse for training. Working with Polly at Lincoln Elementary was a truly fulfilling learning experience. She was a great trainer.

The school district covered their own campuses—three elementary schools, a middle school, and a high school—as well as two Catholic high schools and three Catholic elementary schools.

What a unique experience! The paperwork and policies were all different from what I was used to. I loved working with little ones—and even the teens. To prepare for this new venture, I researched childhood diseases, including the annoying issue of head lice.

Within my first week, I had to help Polly check students from three classrooms for head lice: Put on gloves and pick through the hair to check for the bugs. If you find even one, the child had to be sent home. We did not make too many parents happy with that call. The teachers were also checked for head lice.

One of our local pharmacists told me to rinse my hair with apple cider vinegar as a preventive, because the lice were repelled by the smell.

I was assisting the next day as well, and the teachers had also rinsed their hair with vinegar. One said, "It is worth smelling like a salad not to have lice!"

One male child came back to school the next day after being sent home with lice.

He snugged his little snow hat down over his ears. "Mom says my hat will keep the bugs from going on anybody's head."

Oh, no. I called his mother. "Did you at least use the prescribed shampoo?"

"Ew. No. The hat will do."

"Ma'am, the hat will *not* do. You have to pick up your son and complete the hair treatment as prescribed for lice."

She was not happy, but she did it.

Nursing, Yes I Do!

The most common occurrence in the elementary school nurse's office was "tummy aches." Some children came with just an ache, some with a fever, and some with vomiting. Vomit had to be cleaned up with a special kit as well as disinfectant spraying of the room. In spite of this, that odor could linger for a while.

Splinters were also common, and I got to be a pro at removing them.

I also had an opportunity to work alongside Yolanda at Cleveland Elementary, and that was a different experience. She may have been a great school nurse, but she was a very unusual person. She had more than seventy animals at her home—or at least that's what she said. She included a number of exotic bugs and lizards in the count.

One day we worked together during school physicals, and I had to console her over the death of one of her lizards. I love animals, but I was not quite sure how to manage this. I did the best I could.

Incident reports happened daily. These kids were always hurting themselves. I was sitting at the desk one day at Cleveland Elementary, heard a bang, and then a third-grade boy walked in, holding and rubbing the side of his head.

I said, "Was that your head I just heard banging on a wall?"

"Yes." He never cried.

I took him to the examination room and did a neuro assessment. I got the details about the incident in the gym that had sent him to the office, contacted the gym teacher and the parents, and drafted my report.

The parents picked him up and took him home with the instructions I provided about potential issues with a head injury and when to seek medical attention.

CHAPTER 14 WORKING THREE JOBS

One of the most frequently prescribed medications for school-age children was Ritalin for Attention Deficit Hyperactivity Disorder. The children who needed the medicine would line up at the door for either 10 a.m. or noon medications. I saw a cartoon in the paper once that was so appropriate. It was a picture of a large truck dumping a load of Ritalin in a school parking lot. Certainly, some students, no denying it, were hyperactive. In others the traits were not so obvious, but their physician had officially diagnosed them.

We would have the pills and glasses of water lined up before the Ritalin rush hour.

In one instance, I held out the paper medicine cup with the Ritalin to one boy, like I did with all the other students. Normally the children would open their hands so I could drop the pill in. This child took the medicine cup from my hand and placed it in his mouth with the pill.

I immediately clasped his jaw and lowered his head forward. "Spit it out into my hand."

The other students giggled.

He spit it all out, and the pill was still solid enough for me to use it again. I brought him to the sink. "Open your hand."

He put out his hand.

I dropped the pill in and gave him a glass of water to swallow the pill with.

Middle school students were exhausting with those hormones rushing. Girls experienced their first menses during the school day, was a major traumatic event for them. In rare cases, we had to speak to them about this being a normal process for a girl, because their parents had not. Heating pads were a staple in both the middle and high school nurse's offices.

Nursing, Yes I Do!

The high school student was another animal entirely—the girls with their fashion, hair, and makeup, and the boys with their attitude, posture, and language.

Girls would come to the school nurse's office with cramps, headaches, or in tears because of an argument with a girlfriend or boyfriend.

Boys would usually come in with muscle strains, to be relieved with an ice pack for about an hour. Or they'd have notes with obvious fake parent signatures accompanied by a schmoozing attempt to get out of unwanted classes.

Sore throats were another complaint both girls and boys made to get out of class. Get the tongue blade and flashlight and have them say, "Ahhhh." Nine times out of ten, their throats were fine. I asked one girl to open her mouth, and I had to turn my head away so as not to laugh. It was as if she were the cartoon head on a toothbrush commercial. I never saw a mouth open so wide in all my life!

After I had worked in schools in for a few months, I was sent to Cleveland Elementary on the first day of school to fill in for their school nurse. I arrived and sat down at the desk. I heard someone cry but could not see anyone until I stood up from my chair.

There was a darling little boy who appeared to be a new kindergartner. As I made my way around the desk, I asked, "What is the matter?" As I looked down, I saw what the problem was: He had wet his pants. "Oh, I see, this must be your first day of school. Let's get you a clean dry pair of pants."

Every elementary school nurse's office had a closet of clothes just for such issues. I let him change himself in the bathroom, placed his wet clothes in a bag, and gave them back to him.

If a child was in the office with a significant issue, I called the parents. In this case, the matter seemed obvious and not serious. However, at the

CHAPTER 14 WORKING THREE JOBS

end of the day, this little boy's mother called me, frantic. "What did the school do to him? He has not wet his pants in years!"

I was as calm as I could be. "The first day of school can often do that to children. It is a very new experience."

She hung up on me.

Just in case she reported me, I informed the principal about the matter. Fortunately, she chuckled. "This happens quite a bit, so don't worry."

At the contracted all-boy high school, the gym teachers were called *coaches*, and they held quite a bit of influence. If a boy brought in an excuse to get out of gym, it had to be cleared with the coach. Most times, after I asked the student to wait until the coach cleared the excuse, the student would say, "Never mind," and run out of the nurse's office.

The exam room had a three-feet-high barrel filled with ice packs—trust me, they were regularly used with the number of sports activities at that school.

One morning I walked into the nurse's office and heard a noise in the exam room. When I investigated, I found a student standing on the scale in his tighty whities.

I snickered and then cleared my throat. "Are you feeling ill?"

"No, I'm just weighing in for the wrestling team."

I just nodded. "Okay, continue."

Covering the all-girl Catholic high school was boring. They only had a nurse in the afternoon to covered for the nun while she attended mass. As I walked in on my first day, a very pleasant elderly nun greeted me. She introduced herself, took my hand, and said, "Let me take you to the infirmary."

191

It looked like an old-time infirmary, from the white metal and glass door medicine cabinet to the stacks of clean sheets, single cot, and tiny wooden desk and chair. Of all the times I filled in there, I believe I had only two students, each time for menstrual cramps. If a student needed medicine, this primarily happened in the morning, and one of the nuns marked it in the medication log. These girls were apparently very healthy and truthful.

The three Catholic elementary schools were covered by one of our district nurses three mornings a week. A few teachers were nuns, but all members of the office staff were laypeople. Any medication that had to be administered when the school nurses were off was given by one of the office staff. Most of my duties there included keeping up with physicals for the students to ensure they had all their vaccines, physician visits, medications, allergy updates, and the like.

Classroom Time

If I was asked to sub in a classroom, I arrived early to review the teacher's day planner. I enjoyed the science classes, but I was called for some others as well. At those times, I just gave the class a written assignment to be handed in at the end of the class.

At times, I received lovely questions like, "How do I complete this math problem?"

I did my best to help or referred the student to the alternate math teacher after I checked with him or her.

One day, I was called at 9 a.m. to fill in for Spanish because the teacher had to leave due to a headache. I did have three years of high school Spanish, so that was helpful. When I entered the class, I saw why the teacher had a headache. The class was in total chaos.

I tried to remove the noisiest two students and talk to them in the hall, but by that time, these two students had upset the whole class. I called the

CHAPTER 14 WORKING THREE JOBS

principal's office for help. The assistant principal came into the classroom and read the class the riot act. Thankfully, that worked.

When the day ended, I left the room only to be greeted by the superintendent. "How was your day?"

"Fine, thank you for asking." I suspect my facial expression told a different story.

❦

I enjoyed those darling elementary students. I filled in one day for a third-grade class and checked the day planner. It was scheduled to be a real teaching day.

We started with handwriting. Just when I thought I had this in the bag, one student said, "That's not the way Mrs. King makes her uppercase *I*."

Apparently, they changed the way to write an uppercase *I* since I had been in school.

I quickly said, "Your teacher is correct, my way was the old way."

Following this, the gifted and talented students had to leave for a class in another school, so I took them to the hall, and then an office staff member would take them to the main door and finally to the bus.

In the meantime, I did math and science. Just as I finished the science lesson, an office staff member leaned into the room. "Why are you all not visiting the library?"

"Oh. Sorry." *That was not in the day planner!* But I hustled the students together and headed down the hall, following the staff member since I had no idea where the library was.

When library time and reading were completed, we headed back to our classroom. By then our gifted and talented students had returned. It was time for lunch, but one of my little boys started giggling and fidgeting in his seat.

I knelt beside him. "Is something hurting you and making you move around so much in your seat?"

Nursing, Yes I Do!

"No."

"Great, because we are now ready for lunch."

After lunch, it was time for English, spelling, and a bit of geography.

When I arrived home, I collapsed onto the bed.

My experience with a high school American literature class around prom time was interesting as well. We were to discuss the first two chapters of the book *The Scarlet Letter*. I had read this in high school—so, so long ago. Fortunately, the teacher had left specific questions to ask and her expected responses. Because I was always there early, I had time to do a quick read before class.

During the initial discussion time, I was in earshot of a conversation initiated by a female student with another classmate about the color of the garter for her prom dress.

I looked directly at her. "Please pay attention to our class."

After the second time of reminding her to stop talking and pay attention, I chose an alternate method. "Susan has a question about the color of garter for her prom dress."

They laughed. Susan was unflappable.

"Susan," I said, "what color is your dress, and what are the colors you are considering?"

"My dress is black and white, and I was considering either a pink or white garter."

"Class, let's take a vote. Please raise your hand if you think Susan should chose pink."

I took a hand count.

"Please raise your hand if you think Susan should chose white."

I took another hand count.

CHAPTER 14 WORKING THREE JOBS

The majority said pink, so I looked at Susan. "There, your question has been answered so, now we are getting back to *The Scarlet Letter*."

There were no further disruptions.

Then there was that unforgettable student in an American history class. He walked into class ten minutes late and banged his books on his desk. He wore a safety pin through the septum of his nose.

I raised my eyebrows and glared. "How about walking out of this class and coming back in like a gentleman. And why on earth do you have a safety pin in your nose?"

He walked out of the class and came back in much quieter and sat down. I did not get an answer about the safety pin, but really I was not expecting one.

When I learned of an opening for a full-time school nurse, I jumped at the chance to submit an application. My application was accepted, and I was called in for an interview.

First I was assigned a task: to complete a letter to parents informing them that their child has head lice. I was then asked to triage two separate sets of five situations that were occurring simultaneously, while I was working in a school nurse's office.

Following this, I was directed to what I would refer to the Firing Squad. I entered a room with eight people. It is customary for school staff applicants to be interviewed by representatives from all of the school's departments, as well as a parent. Peggy represented the school nursing department. Each panelist had a question for me, and I felt I did rather well—until the athletic director asked his questions. I was told he would be my boss.

"Do you subscribe to a nursing magazine? Please identify a book or article that best describes the job you are applying for, include the source and author, and then give a brief summary."

My jaw dropped. "Yes, I subscribe to the magazine *Nursing*." I provided a brief summary of an article regarding the use of Ritalin in children. "I honestly do not recall the author of the article."

I left feeling somewhat bewildered, as well as drained. I did not feel very confident.

About five days later I received a letter thanking me for coming in but telling me they had decided to hire another candidate. When I learned who the candidate was, I was happy for her, as she truly deserved it. She had worked as a sub for about five years to my three months. I continued to sub for about another year.

Chapter 15

JUGGLING MULTIPLE ROLES

With my working two other jobs in between all this, we experienced moments of craziness in the house. Working for Neil at Chapel Care was like the work I did at HCS—however, I did not have to open new cases rather completed revisits. That way I would not be the case manager, which would be impossible to do while working part-time. Most often, I got a phone call in the morning giving me my assignment so I could head over from home. I had my nursing bag of supplies and blank visit notes at home to facilitate things.

One morning as I was getting my assignment from Neil, my three children were waiting for me to take them to school. They usually took the bus but loved the opportunity to get a ride from mom instead.

While I was talking to Neil, my older son knocked the lunch out of my youngest son's hand. My daughter then knocked my older son's lunch out of *his* hand. Before long, they were stepping on each other's lunches.

While all of this was going on, I was trying to listen to Neil. I finally picked up a wooden spoon and hit the edge of the table for attention and subsequently cracked the spoon.

Unfortunately, my little darlings did not change their behavior.

After I got off the phone, I just glared at my children. "I hope you are happy with squashed sandwiches." I took them to school.

Nursing, Yes I Do!

When I started at Regency Home Care, my caseload was small, but having me do an occasional IV visit gave the manager more time in the office for supervisor responsibilities.

I was introduced to the other staff members and met four other supervisors who were responsible for the non-intravenous cases, which were referred to as the traditional cases. Kira was a stunning dark-haired, dark-eyed woman with a Russian accent. Linda had short wispy dark hair, blue eyes, and a sharp tongue. Caleb was a serious, dark-haired, tall, well-groomed, young man in his thirties. Lewis was much more approachable than Caleb, appeared to be in his twenties, and was blessed with thick, golden-brown hair. Both ladies impressed me with their ability to dominate a conversation with the men if they disagreed with them.

Amanda was the branch manager, and she had a domineering personality without being nasty.

Tricia was the office manager—she and Amanda were like glue. Neither was the type of person to chit-chat. They were strictly business.

Well, at least that was my initial impression.

Finally, I met the director of nursing and almost fell over. It was Meredith, whom I had worked with in two previous jobs. I decided it was fate that we work together and gave her a hug. She hugged me back.

I had a long conversation with Meredith, and she honestly told me I would be asked to fill in night shifts for long-term patients in addition to the IV cases.

Before my employment was official, I had to complete two tests: one on traditional nursing standards of care and the other on IV standards of care. I passed them both.

I told Meredith I was already working two other jobs so I could work a couple of days a week so possibly, two overnight shifts or one overnight and one day. This work would be per diem, and I told them which days I would be available.

CHAPTER 15 JUGGLING MULTIPLE ROLES

I was really trying not to work weekends, but within the first three months, I did so, to fill in work for all three jobs. One of them had to go.

Most of Chapel Care's patients had multiple sclerosis and needed IV steroid infusions. I made my visits, completed my paperwork, and went home. I was more interested in my work at Regency Home Care or the school nurse position, as they offered a more promising future for me. So after about three months, I quit the job with Neil to focus on the school and Regency Home Care.

I had not worked much with disabled children before, so this aspect of the work was a challenge for me. Not only did I have to do research for school nursing but also for care of disabled children. I dealt with children who had diseases such as cerebral palsy, muscular dystrophy, Crouzon syndrome, DiGeorge syndrome, Prader-Willi syndrome, various types of encephalopathy, cystic fibrosis, and spina bifida, to say a few.

One case I filled in on was a nine-year-old girl with a nonspecific type of encephalopathy. She was non-verbal, non-mobile, and only responsive to pain. She had a tracheostomy and was connected to a ventilator. Her nutritional needs were met by giving liquid nourishment via her gastrostomy tube—commonly called a MIC-KEY primarily used in children.

This child had the most beautiful long, black hair, and the mom refused to cut it. She had the nurses wash it every other day. She was also given a sponge bath twice a day. I had to be trained by one of the regular nurses, and one thing she forgot to tell me was to warm the blankets in the dryer ahead of giving the child a bath.

I generally did the night shift but did fill in on a day shift once when she was due for a hair wash. I had given a patient a hair wash in bed when I worked in the ICU, but their hair was not this long. I was asked to give her the sponge bath first, dress her, and wait about an hour before doing her hair.

During the sponge bath, I kept her covered as best I could because I had been told that if she chilled, her oxygen level would drop, and she might go into respiratory failure.

Well, sure enough, her oxygen level dropped, and she struggled to breathe.

Her mom rushed in. "Throw these blankets in the dryer!" she demanded.

I did so quickly and on high heat, and returned and started to ambu her with 100 percent oxygen while her mother wrapped her with blankets we had.

After several minutes, the patient was breathing easier, and mom had returned with the warm blankets and placed them on her.

Even though I had taken care of seriously ill patients in the critical care units, with this episode I felt inept. I apologized profusely to the mother.

Initially, she was upset, but then she sighed. "It's all right; sometimes this happens to me too. We should wait a couple of hours before we do her hair."

When that time came, I had everything ready, placed warmed blankets on her in advance, and put the bed in the correct position. I gave the mom a heads up that I would be starting.

"Okay, let me know if you need me."

I positioned the bucket, poured warm water over her hair, lathered her with shampoo, and rinsed, followed by a quick wrap of her hair in a warmed towel. I was profusely sweating by the time I finished.

Mom came in and handed me the hair dryer and I dried her hair. The mom saw that I had been sweating and just grinned at me.

The physical therapist was scheduled to come in and introduced me to a new technique in massaging her arms and legs, which she called, "Indian Milking." This involves wrapping the hand around the limb and pulling

CHAPTER 15 JUGGLING MULTIPLE ROLES

from the upper joint to the extremities. I still use that method now, as it is so relaxing.

This little girl was constant care. If one had fifteen minutes here and there, that was the time to complete one's nurse's notes. I became one of the regulars, filling in two days a week, and developed a routine with her. If a new nurse was being assigned, I often trained her.

One New Year's Day, I worked a night shift with the girl. Usually, I got the liquid nourishment for the gastrostomy feed from the refrigerator. This time I opened the door to see two jars, very similar in appearance. I picked both of them up. Only one had the proper label. I put the other one back.

After I set it up, the mom ran in. "Which jar did you use?"

I showed her the empty jar. "This one."

She grabbed it and checked the label. "Oh, good." She relaxed. "I put together some cocktails for the holidays. Wouldn't want to get those mixed up!"

The adult overnight cases I had were usually patients on ventilators, so that was primarily respite care. When I arrived, the family or evening nurse gave me a report about the patient.

Sterile technique took on a different role in home care. When I did trach care in the hospital, we had sterile kits with everything in the kit to perform the task. In the home, we had plastic or glass containers and forceps we washed first with soap and water and then sterilized with boiling water. When we removed the inner cannula (tube) of the trach, we placed it in one container with peroxide, let it sit for a designated length of time, then with the forceps placed it in the other container with vinegar, let it sit for a bit, then placed it on a paper towel to air dry and replace it. Having worked in intensive care units, I was accustomed to suctioning tracheostomies, but the equipment and ventilators were different from what I was used to.

Some patients had rubber foley catheters that were reused after being sterilized with boiling water, peroxide, and vinegar. These were only used for intermittent drainage from a bladder that would go in spasms and not fully empty naturally.

The care I provided for patients was generally monitoring vital signs, making body assessments, maintaining ventilator settings, suctioning, doing trach care, administering medication, doing wound or skin care, and repositioning.

Unfortunately, when you are there for eight hours, sometimes you're asked to do other chores, such as laundry, emptying a dishwasher, or sweeping the floor. Some of these cases were labeled as LPN cases, but I did not care because the work wasn't as stressful, it fit my parenting schedule, and ensured that we still had money coming in.

Occasionally, I would fill in at an alcohol or drug rehabilitation center to administer medication, collect blood or urine samples, or breath testing for alcohol levels.

Filling in at rehab was a real eye-opener. I would be assigned to collaborate with a full-time social worker, who would show me the ropes. They only needed staff relief on evening or night shifts, so I did a few of those.

I would first check the medication records to see who needed medications and when. Usually, only a couple of patients needed medications on my shifts. The desk had to be staffed at all times, and the nurse was usually the one to do it. The social worker helped pass dinner trays, and after dinner, the patients might walk the hall or just stay in their rooms. Most evenings were like this, and most of my conversations were with the social worker.

CHAPTER 15 JUGGLING MULTIPLE ROLES

Sunday evenings were busier, as some patients were out on passes for the weekend. When they returned, the social worker and I had to check their bags for alcohol, drugs, and related products. Mouthwash, toothpaste, and—believe it or not, shaving cream—are alcohol products. Shaving cream, when sprayed around the rim of a cup, would drip pure alcohol into the cup. So, this had to be confiscated. Straws, small mirrors, containers of powder, and small squares of tissue-like paper were considered drug paraphernalia.

Each patient out on a pass got a breathalyzer test. When anyone had a reading of 0.1 or greater, I had to make a report for their file and contact the physician on call. The breathalyzer machine was outside the main door of the unit, past the elevator, and down the hall. I had visions of being hit over the head and the patient taking off. Fortunately, that never happened, and all of them came back as 0.00.

The medication room was locked at all times, so I had the keys. There was an outer door to a room that was used to complete blood draws, and then an inner door led to the medication storage room. The second time I filled a shift, I was working at night. I had gone into the inner medication room to set up my medications.

I heard someone in the outer room and saw a patient. In my haste to reach him, I walked out of the medication room with the medications and locked the door behind me.

The patient began to ramble about medication he was not even taking. I carefully urged him to follow me out to the unit. George, the social worker, was at the desk, and he helped me get the patient back to his room.

Later, I realized I had a problem. I could not find the medication room keys. I had to confess. "George, I locked the keys in the med room."

He laughed. "You are not the first one to do this."

Nevertheless, I still felt embarrassed. When the day nurse came on, she was a bit upset, but they had access to another set of keys.

Nursing, Yes I Do!

⚕

On a particular evening shift, we had a little episode with the security guard on the main floor. One cold and snowy evening, a woman knocked on the front doors, which had an outer and an inner set. The security guard opened the inner door, then the outer door.

The woman grabbed the security guard and pulled herself into the vestibule leaving the two of them locked in there. We had a closed-circuit TV with a visual of the front entrance. When we saw the security guard with the unknown female, George phoned the police. Then he went to the front door.

By the time he got there, the police were already there. Fortunately, the woman was merely trying to get warm. The police took her to a shelter and quietly, but sternly, advised the security guard on how he should have managed the situation.

⚕

On another shift, I was working with a social worker named Tamara. While we were at our desk posts, the patient from room four approached us and began talking about how much he missed his alcohol. He claimed his brain was already pickled and enjoyed the euphoric sensation.

He added, "You two are so little; I could jump over this desk and take care of both of you."

The social worker led with her expertise in therapeutic communication, while I sat there feeling my thighs tighten around that uncomfortable stool we had to sit on. Tamara was successful in altering his thought pattern, and he left us alone.

⚕

I was also responsible for filling in as a nursing supervisor at a nursing home called Crystal Manor—this was a job for a Super Nurse with roller skates. I would arrive at my shift thirty minutes early to get the report from the prior shift supervisor.

On my first shift, I had an angel of a supervisor—she not only gave me a report but took the extra time to point out the important parts of the procedure book and warn me of the usual problems, like aides dictating where they want to work, call-offs by staff, what to do when you run out of someone's medicine, handling incidents on residents, and mealtime. I worked a half-dozen shifts and experienced all these problems.

Fortunately, my first day was quiet, and I had time to review the procedure book. My main concern was what to do if a fire broke out. The nursing home had six units with twenty beds on each. Each unit was run by a unit manager who was an LPN and had one or two LPNs with her, as well as two aides.

All these patients needed partial to total assistance with their personal care needs. Moreover, these patients had communication, cognitive, or behavior issues, and quite possibly a combination. All the patients required positioning at least every two hours, skin protectant on all the bony prominences to prevent skin breakdown, toileting or incontinence care every two hours, feeding for meals and snacks as ordered, medication administration, bathing, and dressing. It was not unusual for some of the patients to receive intravenous fluids, intravenous antibiotics, subcutaneous or intramuscular injections, gastrostomy feeds, and special skin care.

A nursing home is also referred to as a skilled nursing facility, indicating that the residents require skilled care involving tasks like these. The adage in the past was if you go into a nursing home, you go there to die. To dispel that definition, the term *palliative care* was adopted. In short, the facility provides care to support and improve the quality of life for individuals with failing health that is beyond cure or a drastic improvement.

Mealtimes were a job for everyone. Most residents ate in the dining room, so all had to be taken out of bed and transported to the dining room.

Nursing, Yes I Do!

Occasionally, some ate in their rooms, usually because of family demands. If only they knew the problem this caused! It took an aide or nurse from the dining room, who could otherwise be helping four or more residents at a time.

One day, the temperature was ninety degrees, and I just wanted to run to the store and buy popsicles for all the residents. Everyone was groggy and crabby. We encouraged everyone to eat as best we could, and then we transported everyone from the dining room to their rooms and into their beds, carefully using a pivot turn transfer or a mechanical lift.

On another day, a staff member summoned me to a resident's room to assist in a therapeutic one-on-one. The resident was a seventy-six-year-old woman who insisted that we discharge her so she could return to her family in Georgia.

She had been born in Georgia and had moved up north at age twenty to work. She later married and had five children. Her husband had passed away the previous year, and all her children lived nearby. Only her extended family was in Georgia. Because of dementia, her distant past was clearer than her recent past.

I spent thirty minutes speaking with her, taking time to discover that she wanted to speak to a specific family member—her favorite cousin. I contacted her daughter, who gave me the cousin's phone number. Eventually, we made a long-distance call to the cousin. The patient spent ten minutes speaking with her cousin on the phone, and that was the perfect medicine for her.

One evening an aide called off from her shift. I had to rearrange the staff to cover her absence. Normally this would not be a problem.

One of the aides who worked on two south on day shift said, "I can work a double if I can stay on my floor."

CHAPTER 15 JUGGLING MULTIPLE ROLES

"Okay, thank you." I requested the aide who would otherwise have been assigned to work the evening shift on two south to work on three south. Unfortunately, she had a hissy fit. "If I can't work on two south, I'll just go home."

"Please have some compassion," I said. "Your co-worker is working a double shift. She'll be more effective if she can work the floor she's used to."

But she insisted she work her usual unit.

The aide who had offered to work the double shift was on her way down the hall and heard the other aide complaining. The two of them exchanged some violent words with each other.

I took a deep breath and walked in between them. I looked at the aide who offered to work the double. "You may return to two south."

I turned and looked firmly at the other aide. "Team playing is how I work. If you will be a team player and go to three south, I will be up to help you. Does that sound like a plan?"

She grumbled and went to the unit.

I did go up and help her get a couple of her residents ready for bed, and she appreciated it.

That same night, a resident had a fall, possibly fracturing a hip. The unit manager and I evaluated the patient and called the family and doctor. The ambulance arrived in fifteen minutes. We transferred the patient to the hospital, where he was admitted.

Another patient spilled hot coffee on herself, resulting in a second-degree burn. Again, the physician and family were called. We treated the burn with Silvadene, which had to be ordered and specially delivered to the facility by a courier.

It took the staff and me forty-five minutes to complete the paperwork for each incident.

I developed a real appreciation for the staff members who worked with skilled nursing for the elderly. They are clearly not recognized enough.

Chapter 16
TRAINING AIDES

Word was out that the Regency Home Care office was relocating. That meant a shorter drive for me to the office in Midtown and infrequent trips to the Northtown and Southtown locations. Our director of nursing, Meredith, whom I loved so dearly, had left her position for health reasons. She was a very private lady and had lost her husband due to a chronic health issue early in their marriage. Subsequently, she had to work full-time while raising her daughter, although she had some help from her elderly parents.

A pleasant-looking woman names Carla replaced Meredith. She had a delightful laugh, so we all thought things would be good. Then, the administration hired a girl to help with office management two days per week and be the after-hours on-call coordinator three days per week. Her name was Cathy, and we realized we had attended the same grammar school.

Finally, there was an opening for an instructor for the aides, and I was asked to take it. It was a part-time position, but that was all right. I would train environmental aides (EA), personal care aides (PCA), and home health aides (HHA) at all three locations. The classes were one-week, two-week, and three-week courses.

The primary difference between a PCA and an HHA is that while both assist with personal care, meals, household chores, and errands, the HHA receives specialized training and can deal with more complex diet regimes, handle simple dressing changes, and take basic vital signs. An EA

CHAPTER 16 TRAINING AIDES

will only assist with tasks involving simple meal prep, household chores, and errands. The patient's needs dictated which type of aide was right for any given situation.

With this opportunity, I needed to reconsider my part-time commitment to filling in at the school district. While my heart leaned toward school nursing, the job with Regency Home Care showed more promise for me. Ethan and I discussed this, but he said he would support me with whatever decision I made.

I decided to go to my favorite place to think—the beach. I could get there in about six minutes. I loved walking in the sand and sitting on the rocks, watching the sunset over the lake. My mind is always clearer and my body more relaxed when I am there. The sound of the water pushing the sand and hitting the rocks is ever so calming. The feeling of the water rolling over my feet and pressing them further in the sand is soothing.

As I sat on the largest rock I could find, I looked to the sky and asked God to help me find the answer. After much pondering and prayer, I decided to concentrate on the job at Regency Home Care, so I did not accept any more shifts at the school.

My first training course was to be at the Midtown location. I met with Sally, the previous instructor who was leaving our company. She gave me all her manuals with cheat sheets and templates for tests. The training for the EA and PCA were not as strict as for the HHA, because the latter would be issued a certificate by the state health department, so they had to meet specific criteria.

I brought the manuals home to study. As weird as it sounds, I could mix and hang multiple intravenous fluids, troubleshoot a ventilator problem, and debride a burn, but I had difficulty developing a strategy to teach an aide how to reinforce therapist training for a patient on how to properly walk with a cane. I watched videos and found diagrams on the internet to help me.

During week one, we covered general information, including agency policies, emergency protocols, following care plans, organizational skills, following a map, expectations when completing household chores, errands, simple meal preparation, and therapeutic communication. I had only one middle-aged woman in my class for the EA position. The remaining eight students were there for the HHA position.

All went well. Most of the questions were about the agency's policies and how to talk to patients.

One student asked, "What do you say when a patient tells you they want to die?"

"Good question," I replied. "First and foremost, do not leave the room. Furthermore, it is easier if you know what is going on with their medical or social situation. But if you are not aware of it, do not ask them."

Either way, I advised them to begin by reaching out to hold the patient's hand. "Often, they will continue talking, so listening is generally what they need." Fortunately, I also had a video on this type of communication, and it was a great supplement to what I said.

After week one, my first EA student had completed the course and was ready to meet with a supervisor and then the coordinator to get her first assignment.

Week two, I focused on assisting with a bath, dressing, skin care, transferring, turning, and positioning in the bed or chair, toileting, ambulation, wheelchairs, mechanical lifts, and accompaniment to a medical appointment. I also instructed this group about common medical conditions for children and adults and commonly used medications.

This group would merely remind the patients to take any medications on their care plan. This week was fun, as we role-played patients and aides and did mock, hands-on care with each other. We put hospital gowns over

CHAPTER 16 TRAINING AIDES

their clothes for the dressing part. The training room was equipped with two hospital beds, a wheelchair, a mechanical lift, a commode, bath accessories, and medication bottles (which contained mints). Trainees would be signed off on each task.

Technology is always changing, so I advised them that the home may have different types of equipment—if so, a supervisor would instruct and sign them off in the community. The written test was twenty-five multiple-choice questions. All of my students passed. I handed each of them a certificate of completion from the agency, and they were then introduced to the supervisors, who spent a few minutes with them. Then they went to the coordinator to get their first assignments.

Week three was more intense. We went into more depth on common medical conditions and commonly used medications, including complications and how to manage them. This group was trained to prepare diabetic diets, set up an oxygen tank or concentrator for the correct flow, and apply a dressing to a stable skin surface.

This week felt like what I went through in my first week as a nursing student. I went through medical conditions such as congestive heart failure, chronic obstructive pulmonary disease, diabetes with and without insulin, seizure disorders, peripheral vascular disease, and types of blood clots. Upon going through the medical conditions, we did more role-playing on how to respond if a complication occurred.

We talked about safe needle disposal. In the home, it was acceptable to dispose of needles in an empty laundry detergent bottle, and the family was to take this to a pharmacy when it was full.

Before teaching my class the proper way to turn on an oxygen tank, I needed to review it myself. I was glad I did.

Nursing, Yes I Do!

I had one-half of the class working on a project in the classroom and the other half with me in the storage room with the oxygen tank. The tank was a small one, and I began with the safety instructions. "You must turn the correct dial first. If you turn the wrong dial first, the tank can take off like a torpedo." I then showed them the proper use of the tank.

My first two students connected the tubing, then opened the gauge and the flow meter perfectly. My third student was much too impatient and opened the flow meter first.

Before I could stop her, the tank was spinning like a top on the floor. My students in eyeshot of the room apparently remembered what I said about torpedoes and ran out of the way. I grabbed the tank and turned off the flow meter. We all sighed with relief, mixed with a bit of nervous laughter.

"Oh my gosh, I'm so sorry." This third student said.

"Well, the class can all take this as a learning experience." I set the tank upright. "Because it validated what I said about safety techniques."

Some replied, "We won't forget this!"

We used an entire day to discuss diabetic and renal diets and how to prepare them. Diabetic regimens include 1,200-calorie, 1,600-calorie, and 1,800-calorie diets. I used the chalkboard and developed meals for each type of a diabetic diet. I was amazed how much food you can eat, even on a 1,200-calorie diet.

When discussing the renal diet, I stressed the main issue is to restrict sodium and fluids. The amounts for each would be listed for each patient and most patients would already have some of their diet plans made out, so the aides simply needed to follow their plan. "No one expects the aide to be a nutritionist," I told them, "so if there is no meal plan, call the office."

CHAPTER 16 TRAINING AIDES

The written test for this course had fifty multiple-choice questions. One of my students missed the passing grade by just two points. This student did well with the tasks and was a hard worker. So as not to embarrass anyone, I told the students to wait in the conference room until I called them in individually. If they had passed, I sent them to meet with the coordinator for their assignment.

Finally, I sat down with my student who did not pass and asked her five more questions. She answered all of them correctly, so I passed her and then sent her to the coordinator.

After their meetings, the students were asked to return to the classroom, where I had a congratulatory cake. I invited the supervisors and the director of nursing to join us so they could meet them.

My next class was in the Southtown office. It was a little over an hour's drive, taking the highway about half of the way and going through the hills and farms the rest of the way. While it may have been a long drive to work, it was relaxing and picturesque. The office was small, warm, and welcoming, with pictures on the wall, many windows allowing the sunlight in, and the cheery smiles of the office staff. But it was still perfectly professional. The client caseload at this location was a quarter of what we had Midtown.

The director of nursing, Kayli, was a real sweetheart. She was around my age and short like me. I was very impressed with her down-to-earth approach to dealing with her staff and patients. She even asked if I wanted to stay at her home at any time I did not want to commute. I declined but thanked her and said, "If there's ever an issue with the weather, I will take you up on it."

They had one full-time supervisor and one part-time supervisor; however, I did not get a chance to meet them. Kayli would give her supervisors reports about the new hires.

Nursing, Yes I Do!

I had only three students. One was attending for an EA position and the other two for PCA positions. The EA student, Fiona, spoke only Spanish. I spoke *un poco* Spanish—not enough to teach her. We did have an agency procedure book and care plans in Spanish. I spoke with my director of nursing, and we decided to have Fiona read the manual and care plans that were available in Spanish and return for training the following week, when Carmella, the coordinator, returned from her vacation.

I then returned, and with Carmella's help, completed a tailored class for Fiona, who did extremely well. She was quickly assigned to work with various Spanish-speaking clients.

Because I had only two PCA students, I completed this course in one week. All their tasks were signed off and written tests completed and passed.

My next class was in the Northtown office. This was also a drive, but just under one hour and mostly highway, until I exited onto a road of many car dealers, then into a quaint village. The office was within a multiunit professional building. I was given a key to open the office.

I was told the parking lot had a two-hour max, but they would allow you to move the car to another space in the lot. Strange set up!

Our unit included one individual office, a training room, and a supply room. I was told the patient load here was even less than at Southtown. Because of the small caseload, the Midtown director of nursing was responsible for covering Northtown as well. They had only one supervisor, who would communicate with the Midtown DON on a regular basis to keep her up to date.

I had six students, all for the HHA position. The office had such a turnover of staff that they were desperate to have a solid HHA staff presence so they could increase their caseload.

CHAPTER 16 TRAINING AIDES

My initial contact was only with the students—no actual office staff. I had a list of my students' names, and we spent the first hour just getting to know each other. The students and I appreciated this time. I knew we all had to move our cars in the next thirty to sixty minutes, so I then presented my outline for the class. "We will finish in three weeks—or sooner if possible."

Someone asked, "How can we do it sooner?" Everyone was interested in this.

"The class is designed to last three weeks," I said, "however the standard class has more students, so we may be able to finish sooner. But it will be no longer than three weeks."

This brought sizeable smiles to all my students' faces.

We took a break while those who drove moved their cars and those who took the bus waited. Then we began our formal instruction.

By this time, I had learned that by paying attention to my students' eyes, I could tell whether they were absorbed, bored, tired, or confused.

Every so often, so as not to embarrass the student whose eyes told me he or she needed help, I would stop and say something like, "This condition"—or task or whatever the issue was— "may be misleading . . ." and I would elaborate with information that might fill in the gap and make the topic easier to understand. If I still saw that confused look, I would then say either, "Please feel free to ask me a question because there are no dumb questions," or "I would be happy to stay after class with anyone who has questions."

One shy nineteen-year-old student looked like she had many questions but was afraid to ask. I waited until after our first test at the end of the first week. As I expected, she got only 50 percent of the answers correct. A score of 75 percent was a passing grade. She was the only one who failed.

215

Nursing, Yes I Do!

I waited until the end of the class to hand out the tests. As she turned over her paper to see her grade, I glanced from the side to examine her expression and saw her eyes get glassy.

Before I dismissed the class, I said, "I can stay after class if anyone has any questions." I hoped my nineteen-year-old would stay, but she did not.

As a matter of fact, she did not return the next day. Her classmates asked about her.

I replied by saying, "I hope everything is all right."

During our lunch break, I called the Midtown office, got her phone number, and called her. Fortunately, she answered the phone. I asked if she was all right.

She replied, "I don't think this work is for me."

For some reason, I felt there really was a great HHA deep inside. "I disagree, and I would be happy to work one-on-one with you as needed."

She started to cry and then followed with a heartfelt story about being pregnant. The father of the baby left her when he found out, but she was still in love with him.

During this call, a students walked into the small office I was using and asked, "When are we going to start?"

I could not stop this conversation now. I wrote a note: *Please ask the class to read pages 1–25 and write down any questions they have.*

She took the note and returned to the classroom.

My phone call took another fifteen minutes, and I felt I had convinced her to return.

When I went back into the classroom, the students with cars had gone out to move their cars. I ran out to do the same and realized I had locked my keys in the car.

This was not turning out to be a good day.

CHAPTER 16 TRAINING AIDES

I called the automobile club to rescue my keys. They arrived after fifteen minutes, and it took them another fifteen minutes to open my door. By this point I had lost about an hour of class time.

I returned to the training room and apologized to the class.

Someone asked if I had spoken with our lost student.

I said, "Yes, and she will be back tomorrow."

They all felt this was wonderful news.

This was such a great class that when our lost student returned, not only did she receive extra help from me, but also the other students were extremely helpful. She passed the next test with flying colors and did extremely well with the tasks.

We got a little ahead and finished two and a half days early.

During that third week, I watched my students—including my previously lost one—grow in their knowledge base and hands-on care. They were clearly ready to move on to greater things.

My next Midtown class was to be held in a satellite office we rented in an inner-city office building. Because we did not use this classroom much, all the equipment I needed, such as the copy machine, personal hygiene supplies, freestanding patient lift, and more, had to be brought up to the third floor. What a struggle.

One of the part-time coordinators helped move the supplies. As we rolled the copy machine into place, she said, "I lost my uterus on Main Street bringing in this copy machine and need to go back down and get it."

I laughed so hard I was in tears.

This class had seven students, two for the PCA level and the others for the HHA level. One day, while I was in the middle of a presentation, three women dressed in their Sunday best interrupted us. They stood on the opposite side of a high counter.

Nursing, Yes I Do!

I stopped mid-sentence. "Can I help you?"

One replied, "We want job."

I walked over to the counter, but before I could say anything else, the same woman said, "We are looking for Kira."

Then I clearly heard the Russian accent. I held out my hand to her and introduced myself.

She shook my hand. "I am Sophie."

I reached for the phone. "I will call Kira." I dialed the Midtown office.

Betty answered the phone and connected me to Kira. After informing her of the visitors, I handed the phone to Sophie. They talked for a while in Russian.

After about two minutes, Sophie handed the phone back to me. "Thank you."

"You are welcome."

They all left. As I walked back to my class, one student said, "Well that was interesting."

The next day, I returned to the Midtown office because I had to pick up the projector for a class. Kira was there, so I asked if the women who had shown up during my class would be in my next class. She said they might be—and they were.

I taught that also in the Midtown office, with just those three ladies. They were completing only the PCA portion of the course. Sophie spoke English very well, while the other two spoke very little English. Sophie, with intermittent visits from Kira, helped translate.

Chapter 17

UNFORGETTABLE PATIENT CALLS

News of Kira getting married soon and leaving the United States to reside with her husband overseas shocked us all. We would miss her.

The firm asked me to leave the training job to become the fourth supervisor. This job would provide me with a full-time position. I asked who would train the aides and was told they would only hire staff that were already trained. Our office manager would train the staff in policy and procedures.

I talked to the other three supervisors—Caleb, Lewis, and Linda—about their roles. They said we would work 8 a.m. to 4 p.m. Monday through Friday, with one week a month to be on call after hours and weekends. That might involve opening a new case, orienting an aide or nurse to a new case, replacing a foley or IV, or filling a shift. If we filled an overnight shift, we would be off the next day. As a perk for being on call, we would get Thursday and Friday off the week after we were on call.

The work was diverse. In the office, we would complete orders for care of the patients, talk to doctors and insurance companies, and troubleshoot problems in the field. In the community, we would visit patients to recertify their care, open new cases, administer intravenous medications, and make supervisory visits of aides or nurses or orient them to new cases.

Nursing, Yes I Do!

When I arrived home, I felt excited about the new position. Ethan was enthusiastic as well.

I accepted the position. The first three months went by without a hitch.

Meanwhile, our marketing person was out there building up our clientele, and we were opening new cases like crazy.

In the office, besides the work we were already doing, we often had to help with other tasks such as answering calls and helping the coordinators fill some shifts. If they were not filled we might have to work them ourselves. Open shifts were listed on a white dry-erase board. The coordinators were Angela, Dana, and Peggy. Linda and I shared one office, while the boys shared another.

Sometimes we also helped with potential new hires—interviewing them or making calls to check references and prior employment.

One day I interviewed a pleasant, attractive young lady seeking a job as an aide. She had her HHA certificate and gave me references for her prior employment as a private pay aide, as well as with an agency.

After we spoke I ran her criminal background check. The report showed that in the past, she had been arrested as a prostitute.

I told Amanda about it. She said, "They are generally good and caring individuals, so do not hold that against her."

I walked away, my mouth hanging open.

We did hire her, and we had no problems with her.

One aide case we had out in the boonies was a very hard shift to fill. The patient was an elderly lady who lived in an extremely unkempt home—a real fire hazard. There was a walkway of about six inches wide from her door to her bed, which sat in the living room. Beyond that, boxes, broken appliances, old pictures, license plates, and a plethora of junk surrounded her.

CHAPTER 17 UNFORGETTABLE PATIENT CALLS

She was very particular about how she wanted things done, and she was also very racist. If an aide of color walked in her home, she yelled, called the person names, and told the person to leave.

If the aide did not complete her often bizarre requests, such as stacking items in her hallway further blocking a pathway, washing her dishes in cold water, and doing her laundry in the bathtub to say a few, she would insist the aide leave no matter what the person's skin color. The added problem was these aides often did not have their own transportation, so we would cab them there or drive them there and back ourselves.

Linda and I discussed the problem and decided it might be best if we filled the shift ourselves.

We then found ourselves completing tasks such as washing her dishes, sweeping her floor, or going to the grocery store.

One time when I was there, the patient asked me to return a bag of bulk cookies Linda had brought the day before.

She said, "Linda bought the wrong cookies."

"It's not possible to return bulk cookies," I told her, but she just argued with me for several minutes. Finally, I took the cookies and headed to the store.

Obviously, I did not exchange them, but I did buy the cookies she wanted. When I returned, I gave her the cookies, and she said thank you.

Between the two of us, Linda and I filled that shift ten times over two months.

One morning, Angela received a call from the client's son. His mother had called him the night before, talking pure foolishness. When he arrived, he found her unresponsive and not breathing. Angela offered condolences on behalf of all of us.

The supervisory visits for our aides were always entertaining. Aides were to follow a care plan that would include tasks such as assisting with

221

personal care, meal preparation, feeding, reminding the patient to take medications, doing household chores, running errands, and accompanying patients to a medical appointment. They could not drive the patient, as that was a liability, but could accompany them in a cab or meet the service van at the medical appointment.

Sometimes I would find out later that the aide had taken the patient's car and driven them to the doctor as well as the store. Oh, the times, I would have to sit and remind these aides not to drive the patients!

Then there were the aides who would scrub the patient's house like they were from a housekeeping service. I walked in to see one of our aides pulling everything out of the kitchen cupboards and scrubbing them with Murphy's Oil Soap.

"That is not on the care plan," I said.

She replied, in her native accent, "I was brought up to work hard."

At that, I wanted to bring her home to clean my house.

Another hard-working and dedicated aide said to me once, in the middle of applying makeup to a female patient, "I love my job. I sacrificed my marriage for this."

How do you respond to that? I just said, "We're so grateful to have you."

Cathy, my prior grammar schoolmate, was filling in as office manager twice a week and on-call coordinator three days a week for about six months, but she became untrustworthy. When on call, she provided a totally different version of happenings reported by supervisors, to make herself appear as a problem solver. In fact, her stories were all lies.

Amanda caught on to this, and Cathy was fired.

Moreover, Carla was not doing well as our director of nursing. She was not proving to be a mentor, a good resource person, or support to the nursing supervisors. So after only six months, she was fired as well.

CHAPTER 17 UNFORGETTABLE PATIENT CALLS

Carmen, a tiny, well-dressed, middle-aged woman, was hired to fill in for Cathy as on-call coordinator. Amanda decided she did not need a part-time office manager. Tricia was doing a good enough job on her own.

Megan was our salesperson. I did not officially meet her until several weeks after I started in supervision. She was a tall, slender woman with dirty-blond hair whom I would refer to as "Miss Regency." She was a truly devoted company person and really did help us grow.

Bonnie was hired as our new director of nursing. She was a middle-aged woman with short auburn hair who always wore suits. She was a bright lady and delivered what Carla had lacked as a mentor, resource, and support person.

The calls we received never ceased to amaze me. One patient called and said his aide was vacuuming in her bra.

When I called her for an explanation, she apologized. "It is just so hot in this apartment."

"Please come into the office," I said, "and we can discuss alternative attire."

Another strange call came from one of our aides. "I just walked Mr. J. down the street in his wheelchair to meet some people in a car on the corner."

"Was this a problem?"

"Mr. J. asked me to carry a box and hand it to the people at the corner of the street. I did not know what was in the box until they opened it, and I saw guns. There was an exchange of the box for money, and Mr. J asked me not to say anything about it."

I was not sure how to respond to this. *My aide was an accomplice to a felony!* I took a deep breath to stay calm. "Just relax, we'll take care of it."

I went to Bonnie for guidance. The aide was obviously afraid for her life. "I'll discuss this with Amanda. We'll take care of it."

Nursing, Yes I Do!

I never heard another word about it, although the aide continued to serve that client.

When I was offered the supervisory position, I didn't expect the job to include being a chauffeur, but it did. Most of our aides did not have enough money to own a car, so they either walked to cases that were nearby, rode the bus, or took a cab paid for by the company. We drove them if they were otherwise going to call off.

I was at a wake one evening when I was on call. My pager went off, cueing me to report to the on-call coordinator, Carmen.

"Our nursing student aide called off because her car broke down."

"Can't she get a cab?" I asked.

Carmen sighed. "She won't take a cab because her grandmother won't let her."

"Really, I have heard everything!" After venting my frustration about this to Carmen, I said, "I'll call her myself."

This aide was attending a nursing school, and we had a contract to use their students for aide assignments. When I called the aide, she reiterated what Carmen told me. "My grandmother won't allow me to take a cab to the client's."

"May I speak to your grandmother?"

She came to the phone. I explained that the client's home was in the suburb not far from their house. "Will you please let her take the cab? It's only about fifteen minutes."

"Absolutely not." The grandmother would not budge.

"All right. I am at a wake, but I will pick her up in the next fifteen minutes." I am sure my tone was gruff.

"No need to be snippy," the grandmother told me. "You should be more understanding."

CHAPTER 17 UNFORGETTABLE PATIENT CALLS

"Yes, I am thinking about our patient who is waiting for her aide."

When I arrived at the aide's home, fortunately, she came out right away, and we headed to the patient's home. The shift for the aide was 8 p.m. to 11 p.m., and it was already 9 p.m. by the time I got her there. Carmen had already notified the client that the aide was detained.

I dropped off the aide and advised her I would be back by 11 p.m. to drive her back home.

When I returned to pick her up, I decided to give her a pep talk and asked about her interest in the nursing profession.

She answered, "Yes, I like it very much."

"Great, we need caring and dedicated nurses in the field." I added, "If you are employed in a hospital, you must realize if you have a car problem, your supervisor will not pick you up and they will not pay for your transportation, either."

Well, I paid for that statement, because the next day, Bonnie came into my office and sat on my desk. "I got a call from the nursing school. They said you were verbally abusive to one of their students. What happened?"

I told her the story.

"I hear your frustration," Bonnie said, "but your comment was not appropriate."

"I thought I was giving her good advice for her future!" I put my head in my hands. "Ugh, I thought I was being respectful." I looked back up again. "But lesson learned. Thanks."

This little darling aide called off again a couple of weeks later, saying she was sick. She never took another case.

We had several pediatric cases, and one early morning, Carmen called me with a request from one of our LPNs to relieve her at the home of a child with a seizure disorder by 7:30 a.m. so she could get to her other job

Nursing, Yes I Do!

at the school. I arrived about five minutes late because of traffic and found the nurse waiting for me outside, fuming.

I got out of the car. "I'm sorry I'm late. It was out of my control."

She headed toward her car.

"Wait, you need to give me a report! And where is the child?"

"On the sofa."

"You left a two-year-old, developmentally delayed child *with a seizure disorder* on the sofa unattended? Please follow me so I can check on the child and hear your report."

Trudging behind me she muttered, "You know, I do *not* have to fill in these shifts if I don't want to."

After I checked on the child, the LPN gave me a two-minute report and left.

When I returned to the office later that day, Bonnie came to see me again. She said this nurse was threatening to quit because of my comments.

I gaped at her. "I am truly sorry, and with all due respect . . . I am getting confused about what the real definition of responsibility is with our staff."

With pursed lips, Bonnie took a deep breath. "You are correct. But as management, we must be compassionate to both the staff and the patients. Next time, leave the disciplining to me. I will take the bullet. Feel free to come and talk to me first when you feel frustrated with irresponsible staff members. That way we can support each other."

I agreed.

Opening cases was always a long process. I received a call in the office to open a case on a set of triplets. They had jaundice, a condition common in newborns. Bilirubin, a compound that is normally broken down and excreted in urine, can build up in the body and cause yellow skin discoloration. It is easily treated with bili lights, which emit a blue light that helps

CHAPTER 17 UNFORGETTABLE PATIENT CALLS

the body break down the bilirubin. In addition to that, these triplets also had apnea, a breathing disorder, so they were on oxygen, with monitors to check for abnormal heart rhythm and blood oxygen levels. They also required a bilirubin test in the morning. I made my initial visit to the BAS Pediatric Center and assessed each of the newborns, received orders for each, and developed a chart for each of them.

That evening, I was to meet one of our staff registered nurses, whom I would train to serve the newborns. On arrival at the home, I met the mom, who led me into their family room where the three little darlings were lined up in their bassinets under the blue lights. They had just arrived home about an hour before.

A nurse from BAS Pediatric Center had followed them home to set up the oxygen and monitors. Melody, our RN, arrived two minutes after me. She and I introduced ourselves and reassured the mother of our experience with babies. Then we walked over to the newborns.

I pulled out the charts, and Melody and I checked the names on the wristbands of the newborns and reviewed the orders.

"Oh, the oxygen settings and amount of nourishment are different for each of them," Melody said.

The mom just stared at us for the first couple of minutes. After hearing us talk medical lingo and seeing us checking everything carefully, she appeared to relax.

I turned back to her. "Melody will be here from 7 p.m. to 7 a.m., and Sandra will cover the 7 a.m. to 7 p.m. shift. Melody will return at 7 p.m. for another twelve-hour shift."

The mother nodded.

"If the babies' blood levels and oxygen levels are stable, Sandy won't *have* to come back again the next morning, but I recommended having her come back anyway. If things are good, she can leave early."

Nursing, Yes I Do!

"Oh, that sounds great, thank you!" The mom seemed happy that I was taking the extra caution for the benefit of her babies.

When Sandy arrived that second morning, she discontinued the oxygen, as ordered by the pediatrician. She used pulse oximetry to monitor the babies' oxygen levels on room air. The pediatrician had advised us that if the oxygen levels reached a certain level, we could discontinue home care services.

Their oxygen levels were good on room air, and Sandy was able to go home by noon. Our office received a beautiful thank you card from the family.

I'll never forget Ms. Z. She was a thirty-five-year-old multiple sclerosis patient. She was already on twenty-four-hour LPN service when I started with the company.

Originally, her daughter lived with her, and we provided an aide for just two hours per day.

Over time, Ms. Z's needs increased. She required a nurse because of routine straight catheterizations to drain her bladder of urine and range of motion exercises met by a daily visit. We tried to teach her daughter how to perform a straight catheterization and range of motion exercises, but she refused to learn and subsequently moved out.

Considering that Ms. Z required twenty-four-hour supervision, we recommended placement in a skilled nursing facility. She refused and, with her attorney's assistance, we were forced to put in twenty-four-hour care, most of which was nursing. The attorney arranged for her brother to take care of any plumbing, electrical, and other household maintenance responsibilities.

In the office, it was not unusual to see her name on the open shift list on the dry erase board. Filling her shifts was difficult because she was so hard to deal with, for multiple reasons. For example, when you performed the

CHAPTER 17 UNFORGETTABLE PATIENT CALLS

straight catheterization, she would talk you through the procedure, stressing how to cleanse her and where her urinary opening was. She spared no details. Then she'd sigh with relief when you passed the catheter in.

Ms. Z had to be transferred out of bed to her electric wheelchair after her bath in the morning, and since she was about 160 pounds, this was a bit of a challenge for one person. I was convinced she had a demon in her because she would make it harder by pulling on the rails on the opposite side.

I transferred her several times with no problem; however, one time, she pulled so hard against my efforts that she almost fell. In preventing her fall, I threw my back out, causing me to lose three days of work.

She insisted on taking a sleeping pill every night. Her standing instruction to the nurses was that if she were asleep at 11 p.m., they should wake her up to give it to her.

At night, she would usually give you instructions to complete tasks such as doing the laundry, washing dishes, sweeping the floor, or cleaning her refrigerator. She would often hit, slap, pinch, or punch the nurses if they did not follow her directions. The directions for these tasks would change frequently, just to allow her to be in more control. She also criticized you the whole time you were there.

As a nurse, you are supposed to just tune out the negatives, because your patients are ill. However, as a human being, your patience often runs thin. I would try to find some humor in it.

One night I was filling the 11 p.m. to 7 a.m. shift. The nurse I was relieving said, "She has been sleeping since 10 p.m. and I really must go home. Would you mind walking her up for her sleeping pill?"

"Of course not."

After she gave me her report, I walked into the bedroom, where the patient was sound asleep. I knew she would yell at me if I did not wake her to give her the sleeping pill so, with a flashlight in my hand, I waved the

Nursing, Yes I Do!

light around the room in a silly manner while calling out her name in an attempt to wake her.

She did not awaken. On assessment, I found she was breathing fine and had a good pulse, so I went back to the kitchen.

After two hours, I heard her voice, "Get in here right now."

I entered the bedroom.

"Where is my usual nurse?"

"She is ill."

"You should know, I needed my sleeping pill at eleven o'clock, and you were supposed to wake me."

"I tried. But you were sleeping so soundly, I let you sleep."

"That was not your decision."

"How do you recommend I wake you?"

"Just call my name."

There was no sense going further with that, so I returned to the kitchen where her medications were stored and brought back her sleeping pill.

She grabbed my arm and almost pulled it out of the socket.

The pill dropped to the floor.

After she let go of my arm, I looked at her as if I were her mother. "I am going to the kitchen. When you are ready to behave like an adult, I will return with another sleeping pill for you."

Her mouth dropped open. It took her fifteen minutes to call me back, and she was quiet the rest of the night.

Chapter 18

DRAWING A LINE

Caleb, Lewis, Linda, and I were filling shifts a couple times per week. We compared notes. Some nights, we had more than one open shift, and whichever of us was on call would have to call one of the other supervisors to fill the extra shift.

We were all salaried employees, so the shifts we filled were "bill no pay." That is, the client was billed but we were not paid anything above our regular salary for filling those shifts.

"The company must be making out like a bandit," Caleb said.

Linda nodded. "Yeah, it looks like we're being taken for granted."

"It's true," I said. "This has to change."

We all decided that the next time there was more than one open shift, we would advise the director of nursing that no other supervisor was available.

One day, after starting work at 8 a.m., I completed my office work and prepared to take call after the office closed at 5 p.m. until 8 a.m. the next morning. I had to open a new case by 6 p.m. This took me three hours. The patient was a young guy just getting out of the hospital after back surgery. His case was complicated by a need for IV antibiotics every twelve hours. He needed an aide to help him get ready for bed that night and an aide in the morning for his bath and dressing.

Nursing, Yes I Do!

I started his IV antibiotics at 8 p.m. and trained the aide to fill the shift. I already knew I had to fill another overnight shift for Ms. Z from 11 p.m. to 7 a.m. I had time to grab a bite to eat and change my clothes. I always kept a bag in the car with comfy clothes in case I needed to fill a shift when I was on call.

While I was on Ms. Z's shift, Carmen called. A cancer patient was being discharged in the morning, and I had to open that case and give her IV chemotherapy.

I headed to my IV antibiotic patient at 8 a.m. That appointment took an hour. After that, I headed to my new case to administer IV chemotherapy—that took two hours.

While I was at my IV chemotherapy case, Carmen called again. "I had to fill an open shift at an aide case, and I will need you to orient the aide."

I accepted the extra task and then added, "After this, I am signing off to Bonnie, because by the time I get home, I will have been working thirty-four hours."

When I got home, I called Bonnie and told her briefly how my night had gone. "I can't keep my eyes open any longer. I need to go to bed."

"What about Caleb, Lewis, or Linda?"

"They're unavailable." This was stretching the truth because I hadn't actually talked to them that day. But that was the agreement we had reached.

When I woke up, I wrote a full summary of my travels and tasks for the previous night so I could give it to Amanda.

On Monday, I met with her and presented my summary and the number of hours I had to stay awake. "I will never do this again."

Her eyes popped open. "Yes. I'm sorry. That shouldn't have happened."

CHAPTER 18 DRAWING A LINE

When I left Amanda's office and headed to mine, I felt the eyes of Caleb, Lewis, and Linda on me—they must all have been wondering what Amanda said.

I approached Linda. "It's all good. We can talk about it at our weekly team meeting on Wednesday."

Bonnie and Amanda did not always attend that meeting, but they did so this time. We discussed the extended shift I had undergone and came up with a plan to avoid having that happen again.

"What we need," Bonnie said, "is a written statement from any supervisor who's called to assist another if they're unable to do so and why."

Amanda was quick to add, "We don't expect all four of you to be always on call. If you're unreachable on the days you're not on call, I support that."

Both of them endorsed what I had done, but just wanted to document the discussion. They also implemented a policy of refusing a new case after our usual office hours if the on-call supervisor had already worked more than twelve hours.

Office Party for the Children

Once a year, our three offices collaborated to have a party for the disabled children we served. This was my first time participating, so I looked to my peers for guidance on how this was done. The menu included pizza, subs, cake, and soda, and we also had games and activities for the children and their families. Since ours was the larger of the three offices, the party was held there. It was nice to see Kayli, the director of nurses from the Southtown office, again.

We were allowed to bring a family member to help. My daughter, Aurora, was eleven, and I thought this might be a good experience for her. Amanda's daughter was the same age, so they worked together on a coloring activity with two of the children. Aurora was afraid initially, but as soon as she got

233

a little response from the child, her fear passed. Watching her communicate with this nonverbal child through art gave me a warm feeling throughout my body. She would never get an opportunity like that in school.

All in all, it was a great event and well attended by about twenty-five children and their families. The parents were extremely appreciative. After the families left, Megan brought out some champagne and poured a glass for each employee. After an hour of cleanup, I needed to get my exhausted little girl home.

On the drive home, she asked around twenty questions about disabled children, but soon she was sound asleep. Looking at her in the rearview mirror sleeping so soundly just made me smile. I hoped she would always remember that experience.

Expanding the Business

Megan had been very busy getting contracts for more work. One of these was with the Cancer Research Institute. We would follow their patients at home and administer supplemental IV chemo, vitamins, antibiotics, or just IV hydration, as well as continuing assessments and patient teaching.

The discharge planner, Lucille, was our primary contact, but she had very little faith in us. She was intimidating and critical, saying things like, "If your pharmacy does not deliver the medications on time, we will cut the contract with you," and "I know you may find this hard to understand, but you must follow our diet plan for the patients."

I had never met this woman before, but she spoke like this to all of our staff. Rumor had it she wanted a company called IV Guard to take the full contract; instead, a split contract was made between us.

Caring for cancer patients was another challenge. It was not unusual to find your patient bald, pallid, and vomiting during a visit. Foods recommended for these patients were canned fruits and vegetables and soft meats, as they were more palatable and easier to digest. Keeping the patients

CHAPTER 18 DRAWING A LINE

hydrated was very important. Plain water is insufficient in such cases, so we used Gatorade or Pedialyte. On hot days, we made popsicles for them. It was often hard to leave these patients' homes because they often needed extra time just for reassurance.

Evgeni was a male patient, nineteen years old, of Slavic decent, who was living in the area to attend school. He had been in this country only eighteen months when he was diagnosed with leukemia, a cancer of the blood-producing system. His father and brothers flew to the United States to be with him during his treatments. They stayed at the local Ronald McDonald House.

I was scheduled to give him IV chemo, and the medication he received was flown in by helicopter. I arrived at the house as scheduled and met him and his family. This was during midwinter, and an intense snowstorm delayed the helicopter that day.

Evgeni's dad was preparing dinner and insisted that I join them. I have learned that you never refuse when Europeans offer you food, or they will be insulted. So, I said thank you and enjoyed a delicious meal.

The medicine finally arrived two hours late, and I administered it via his central line. I said my farewells to him and his family, which included a hug, and said I would return in three days for his next infusion.

The following day in the office, Megan asked, "What happened with the IV chemo for Evgeni? Lucille called and was ready to pull the contract."

Knowing Megan was a great negotiator, I said, "I'm sure you talked her out of it."

"Well, yes, but—"

"The weather was horrible," I said. "That affected the delivery time."

She frowned. Regency Home Care was a national agency, and our pharmacies were located sparsely.

Nursing, Yes I Do!

I added, "If we had a local pharmacy, this might not have been an issue."

She knew there was nothing to be done about it because she said nothing else and walked back to her office.

I gave Evgeni his chemotherapy supplement for three more sessions. Before his fourth session, I learned he had taken a turn for the worse. He'd been admitted to the Cancer Research Institute and passed away.

We were all saddened in the office. Megan sent a bereavement card to the family on behalf of the agency.

As nurses, we are supposed to be able to separate ourselves emotionally from our patients so our relationships with them do not interfere with our judgment. I can do that while they are still alive. But when they pass, it is as if that program in my head gets turned off, and the reality of the end of life takes over.

When I arrived home that evening, I was not hungry. I asked my husband to tend to the kids so I could go to bed. I fell asleep as soon as my head hit the pillow.

Another contract Megan signed was with a pharmaceutical company to administer a drug known as Flolan. This was to treat Class III and IV pulmonary hypertension (extremely high blood pressure). Patients had a very limited life expectancy without this drug. Candidates for this drug had to be mentally alert and cognitively able to self-administer this lifelong treatment with an able and willing secondary caregiver. The infusion would run for twenty-four hours, seven days per week. In other words, nonstop for the rest of their lives.

The medicine was packaged in cassettes, and each patient would get either one cassette to run over the full twenty-four hours or three eight-hour cassettes, requiring changes three times per day.

CHAPTER 18 DRAWING A LINE

The company brought in their trainer to educate us on this drug and how to train patients. Linda, Caleb, Lewis, and I had one full day of training, which I found very interesting. Apparently, my interest showed. The corporate representative asked me to be the trainer representative for our eight-county region, and my peers were relieved to not have that responsibility.

Because I was chosen, I needed one more day of training. Amanda and Bonnie were happy for me and said they would re-assign some of my supervisory cases. To keep insurance costs down, I was to provide teaching on this regime in three visits. The insurance would pay for a portion of the drug, and the patient had a somewhat large co-pay, so my patients were apparently of the higher middle class and up.

My first patient was a retired saleswoman for a prestigious company. She had taken a stimulant years before to lose weight. Research has shown that this drug may cause a person to develop pulmonary hypertension.

When I arrived at the home, her husband answered the door and led me into their kitchen. "My wife will be down soon. She never comes down until she is *fully* dressed."

Mrs. Y entered the kitchen, fully dressed, including full makeup. She was an attractive middle-aged woman; however, I could see the fear on her face behind the fake smile.

I shook her hand and introduced myself. We made small talk for about ten minutes. I grabbed the first possible segue to begin my training. The box of supplies was on the table. "I need to make sure we have all the supplies before I begin." Fortunately, everything was there. She had been issued one cassette for every twenty-four hours.

I laid all the equipment on the table. "I realize this may look like a lot, but once we review all the pieces and go over the steps, you'll see this is fairly elementary."

Nursing, Yes I Do!

Mrs. Y and her husband were quick studies, and they might have been okay after just two visits, but I felt more comfortable going the third day, especially since this was my first case. On day three, when I bid my farewell, Mrs. Y hugged me and cried. I comforted her a few minutes, wished her the best, and headed out the door.

My second patient was Mr. X, a young gay fellow who was HIV positive. This, too, is a trigger for pulmonary hypertension. When I arrived at his home, I found him to be a very thin, sad, young man. I began with small talk about my drive over. Seeing he was not interested, I jumped into the start of my training, checking the supplies, laying them out, setting up the cassette—talking the entire time with some participation from him.

He watched me with total amazement and performed his piece of the task appropriately. He asked, "Will this keep me alive?"

"Yes, that is the plan, provided you have no other complications."

He sighed. "I should have known the answer. Nothing is for certain."

This was my segue to discuss his emotional status. "Do you think you might benefit from counseling?"

"Yeah, probably."

I made a note. "I'll contact your doctor to make some arrangements. You and I can talk more about this when I return tomorrow."

He smiled. "Thank you."

After I left, I phoned the doctor and spoke at length about Mr. X's emotional state.

The doctor said he would contact a peer who made home calls. "I'll call Mr. X to fill him in."

I found that a relief.

When I returned the next day, the psychologist was just leaving. We shook hands and introduced ourselves.

CHAPTER 18 DRAWING A LINE

I entered the room where Mr. X was and said, "Are we ready to begin today?"

"Yes. Thank you for the quick help. I appreciate it."

"You are so welcome."

He was in a much better mood. That day and the next flew by. When the time came to bid farewell, I got another hug and some tears before I finally left.

My next patient was Mr. W. His pulmonary edema was more severe and required three cassettes per day. He was an overweight, middle-aged man with lung disease. He would huff and puff to regain his breath after minimal exertion.

Fortunately, he had two daughters to assist him and learn the technique of the cassette changes. They struck me as very dedicated, but worried, young ladies.

I took my time explaining the process. Three times during my instruction, I asked if they had any questions or concerns.

One of them asked, "What would happen if Dad were hospitalized?"

"Don't worry about that." I showed them the label on the side of the cassettes. "These all have the contact information to call the pharmacy or our agency. We would take it from there."

Mr. W. had some difficulty performing the task, but his daughters helped him out. After three days, I had one more signed off.

About a month later, our receptionist advised me that the wife of a veteran with Class IV pulmonary hypertension had called.

When I called the wife, as soon as I said hello, she burst into tears. "Will a nurse come to our house three times per day to change these cassettes?"

Nursing, Yes I Do!

Lucky me to get this call. "Ma'am, we can only provide teaching to the patient and one or two caregivers. From there on you'll need to complete the changes."

"I can't!" She continued crying. "I cannot learn this... I'm too afraid."

"Is there another family member or friend—preferably two—who could help?"

Her voice squeaked. "No."

Our conversation went on for forty-five minutes, and I could not terminate the call on this frantic woman.

Finally, I referred her back to the doctor. "You can ask whether he has another plan. Or you can reach out to other veterans."

This quieted her down some so I could end the call.

Chapter 19

FAMILY TROUBLES

Amanda was out of the office for a three-day conference. On one of those days, Bonnie called in sick—highly unusual, as she was always so healthy.

Of course, the shit hit the fan.

One of my aides called in a panic. She was providing personal care help and meal prep for a seventy-five-year-old woman I'll call Mrs. V. Mrs. V lived with her two adult sons. One son, Gordon, was developmentally challenged, unable to help his mother other than doing some basic housekeeping. The other son, Bert, had a history of mental illness and inability to help care for his mother. Bert lived in the back apartment, which was fine if he had stayed there. Whenever he did present himself to one of our aides, he made them nervous.

On this occasion, Bert had come out, grabbed a frying pan, and chased our aide. The first time our aide called she uttered only about five words and hung up, so I had no idea who it was.

The next time she called yelling, giving her name, the name of the client and followed with, "The son from the back apartment came out . . . he is chasing me with a frying pan . . . his brother is trying to protect me."

Although we knew Bert had a mental illness, because of HIPAA protections, we weren't told what. Based on his behavior the few times we had seen him, we guessed that dealt with paranoid schizophrenia.

"Stay on the phone with me!" I said. "We'll call the police on another line." I signaled our coordinator, Angela, to call the police to this client's address.

I stayed on the phone with her until the police arrived, and then I asked to speak to the officer.

The officer took the phone, and I asked, "Do you think our aide is in any danger?"

"There's no injury," he said, "so I can't arrest the son, but I advise you to have the aide leave the house."

I relayed that information to the aide and then asked to speak to Mrs. V. Upon hearing her voice on the phone, I asked, "Do you feel safe staying in the house? If not, I can make arrangements for you to be admitted to a facility short-term until we resolve the issue with Bert."

"I'm not leaving my house."

"All right, but I must tell you that we will not send another aide there until Adult Protective Services have intervened."

"I understand."

First I contacted the doctor to update him, and he agreed with me. I followed up with a call to Adult Protective Services (APS) and filed the complaint. I informed them the patient would not receive services until they evaluated Bert's mental health and provided us with a report.

"We might not be able to get out there for three days," the APS representative told me. "You should send the aide to help Mrs. V."

"I offered to have Mrs. V transferred to a facility for her protection, and she declined. If that is your protocol, contact us when you have made the visit and made your determination."

The APS representative groaned and hung up on me.

I was a bit of a wreck as I made this decision without consulting a manager, but we could not reach either of them.

Bonnie's son called later to say she was very ill and sleeping, so we wished her well.

Amanda called back. When I reported the story to her, she fully supported me.

CHAPTER 19 FAMILY TROUBLES

After four days, we received a call from APS asking us to attend a meeting at the county office. Angela accompanied me to the meeting. We sat at a table with the representative from APS, the director of nursing from the County Home Care Program, two caseworkers, and the director of the social services program—who fell asleep five minutes into the meeting.

The APS representative reported going to Mrs. V's home and meeting with five other family members we never knew existed. I wondered if he had the right house. At any rate, he said Mrs. V was having her needs met by these family members.

"What about Bert, the mentally ill son?" I asked.

"I never saw him."

My mouth dropped open. I could not help but say, "That was the whole reason for your visit."

He ignored me. "We must put the aide back in."

"Since you did not complete the evaluation of the mentally ill son, we cannot guarantee the safety of our staff in that home. Contact us when you have." I stood up, Angela and I left.

Now it was their turn to have their jaws drop open.

Angela patted me on the back. "Good work!"

Three days later, I received a call from the APS representative. They had spoken to Bert at length. "We have no reasons for concern."

"I need you to give me that in writing," I said.

"Okay, we'll get a letter in the mail."

As much as I wanted to wait for the letter, it was best for the patient to get an aide back out there.

I arranged to meet the aide there and check the house. On my arrival, the aide was waiting in her car. We approached the front door together. Gordon, the son who lived with the patient, answered the door. He let us in and apologized about his brother. "If Bert comes out again and causes a problem, I'll call the police myself."

He also showed us the door to his brother's apartment. "My uncle put this latch on the door. We can go in to take Bert his food and stuff, but this keeps him from coming into Mom's apartment."

That relieved both of us.

Holiday Snowstorm

On the Friday after New Years' Day, 1998, snow fell on and off all day and was expected to continue for the next couple of days. It was my weekend to be on call. I was just wrapping up my paperwork and everyone else had left for the day. I was about to leave and suddenly felt I needed to do one more thing.

About four months earlier, we had labeled our cases with a triage code of one, two, or three in the event of an emergency. But we had never put an actual list together. I felt today was the day to do it. It was already 6:30 p.m., but I had a feeling I *needed* to do this. It took me about an hour to go through our covered cases to obtain the codes.

I was totally exhausted by the time I got home. Luckily, I did not have to fill any shifts. On Saturday and Sunday, for the two shifts that had call-offs, we were able to taxi substitute aides to the patients. A couple of times, we needed four-wheel drive vehicles.

On Monday we were hit by a megastorm, and most roads in the county were closed. The first call we received was from Dr. U. He and his wife were the parents of a disabled child who was pretty much in a vegetative state. We provided nurses for eight hours during the day and an aide eight

CHAPTER 19 FAMILY TROUBLES

hours overnight. He was in a panic because the aide had called him and said she couldn't get there.

Carmen, our coordinator, said she would take care of Dr. U and explained about the road closures, but he became irate and insisted we send his aide. Out of frustration, she hung up. "For heaven's sake, he's a doctor! Can't he and his wife care for their child during this storm?"

We giggled about the fact they would only accept one particular aide, because she not only re-positioned and changed diapers for their child, but she did the family ironing and prepared their dinner for the next day. That was not on the care plan nor expected of the aide, and our county dollars paid for it.

The next call came from Ms. Z. Of course, she was triage level one, so we had to fill her shift. It almost looked like I would have to fill the shift myself. After I called Amanda to explain the difficulty filling it, she said, "Offer the nurse an extra fifty dollars, because I need you to keep working the phones with Carmen."

That worked. On the next call, I got a nurse to fill it.

I was on the phone so much my ear was perspiring. This continued for twenty-four hours.

Bonnie's Farm

The cold months passed, and we were anxious for June, as Bonnie's daughter was getting married, and we were all invited to the wedding. Ethan was out of town for work, and since our children were invited I brought Aurora and Dominick. Cameron had another commitment.

Unlike other weddings I have attended, this was a very informal wedding in the yard of the farm where they lived. Bonnie had horses and had told me to please bring our children so they could ride. It turned out to be a busy weekend for most of our office staff, so Amanda, with her daughter, was the only other co-worker there.

245

Bonnie had a large farm where she bred horses and maintained a large apple orchard. She had talked before about routinely feeding her horses in the morning before she came into work, and she spent her weekends maintaining the orchard.

She had a small English garden as well. There, Aurora, and Amanda's daughter picked flowers. After the girls discovered that Bonnie's daughter did not have a veil, the girls created a flower veil that she wore when she exchanged her vows with her husband.

After the ceremony we ate, and then it was time to ride the horses and later, dance. My Dominick was so impressed with the horses that he asked me for one all the way home.

The next several weeks were like a whirlwind of work. I could hardly catch my breath.

I stopped at the grocery store after work one Friday evening. As I unloaded the groceries at home, Ethan met me at the car with the phone in hand and a sobering look. "Linda is on the phone. You better take it now. Bonnie passed away."

I gasped for breath. I felt limp and my eyes began to swell. I took the phone and walked into the house. I didn't speak until I had sat on the sofa. "Linda?"

She was sobbing.

That led to my sobbing for a minute. Finally, I said, "How did this happen?"

"Bonnie's daughter said it was a heart attack."

Bonnie had been working in the apple orchard and collapsed. Her two dogs were with her and lay beside her until a driver from the road saw them and called for an ambulance.

She was already gone.

There was going to be a single evening wake for friends and family, followed by a private memorial service. Bonnie was ten years older than I.

CHAPTER 19 FAMILY TROUBLES

At the wake, standing beside Amanda, I looked at Bonnie lying in her casket. "I do not want that to be me in ten years."

Amanda looked at me and nodded.

Moving On

It was hard to believe we needed to replace another director of nursing. But Amy was a real gem—a very pretty lady of about fifty years old with short blonde hair, sky blue eyes, and a feisty personality. She had many years of bedside nursing experience followed by several years as an administrator. When we entered her office to discuss an issue, she always greeted us with a smile. The director of nursing had always evaluated our reports, but Amy was very fussy about these reports, so it was not unusual to get our reports back with a few notes for corrections.

Linda and I had gotten close and shared a lot of our lives. When Linda was stressed, she would develop hives around her neck. I would give her a heads-up when I saw those nasty marks developing.

Sometimes, she would feel it and say, "Is my neck red?"

"Yep, you did it again."

She was five years younger than I and had two children, ages three and five. Linda had an Irish setter, and I would hear stories about Abby all the time. I told her a few times about how much my kids and I wanted to have a dog, but my husband did not and lately was concerned about not having enough time to train a puppy.

Linda's husband got a job transfer to Miami, Florida, and she totally surprised me by asking if we would take Abby. She said the heat in Miami would be too much for her, and she wanted to find a good family for her. Without hesitation, I said yes.

Abby was five years old, so no puppy training would be needed. When I came home that night and told the family, the kids jumped up and down while Ethan just gave me a smirk.

Nursing, Yes I Do!

He soon fell in love with Abby.

I missed Linda, but because we knew she was leaving, Amanda had already started recruiting so I never needed to cover her patients.

Our new teammate, Monica, was a quick study. She was a little older than I, short like me, and had beautiful blonde hair she always kept up in a bun. Her personality was warm and welcoming.

Work remained busy, and I filled many overnight pediatric shifts. Each mom knows best for her child, but when our nurses provided care to their children, the moms had to follow doctor's orders. All too often, mom would have her own orders for medications and treatments and expected our nurses to follow her orders and not the doctors' instructions.

We got used to having to call the doctor when mom's orders conflicted with theirs. Some nurses took the chance and followed mom's orders, while others basically educated mom on their licenses and suggested she carry out the tasks for her own orders.

The most common request made by moms was lifting techniques. Many of our disabled children were eighty pounds or more, and moms would often decline the use of mechanical lifts and request that the nurses carry the child.

I agree that bringing the mechanical lift into a small bathroom to shower a child could be cumbersome. So, I ended up carrying an eighty-pound child from her bed down the hall to the bathroom and placing her in the shower chair.

One mom insisted we transfer her child to and from a sandbag chair on the floor. This child was ninety-five pounds, and we had way too many cases of our nurses injuring their backs. We had to educate the parents on safe transfers—not only for the child, but for the nurse as well.

CHAPTER 19 FAMILY TROUBLES

An Answer to My Prayers

My eldest had graduated from high school but still lived at home, working part time. My younger two both had a lot of activities going on at school and after school. My parents were getting up there in years and needed more help. My work schedule made it difficult to accommodate all of these responsibilities. I pleaded with God to show me a way through these challenges.

Callie, whom I had known as a nurse from St. Christopher's Hospital, called. She was working for a company named Dorm. She had been there for about five years and was very happy. "We have an opening for a nurse."

"What's the job like?"

"The job title is assessor nurse. The primary role is monitoring home care services for Medicaid patients. Mainly observation, interviewing, and documentation."

Sounded like it didn't involve a lot of patient care.

The hours were regular banker hours—8 a.m. to 4 p.m., except one day every two weeks of 8 a.m. to 5 p.m. "Plus you'd have every other Friday or Monday off," she said.

The schedule seemed like a good fit for our family life. "Who do I call for an interview?"

When I arrived home from work that day, the first thing I did was update my resume. The next day during my lunch hour, I called the director of nursing's office and asked if I might send a copy of my resume for the assessor nurse position. A very pleasant lady gave me the address, and I put it in the mail the next day.

I received a call from Dorm five days later and was asked to come in for an interview. I was thrilled, and immediately agreed to an appointment the following Thursday at 9 a.m.

Arriving at the office, I recalled negative memories, because Dorm occupied the same building where I had attended that meeting with Adult Protective Services. This time, I paid more attention to the surroundings.

The building was an old dance hall with unfinished hotel rooms above. The three ballrooms there had been used frequently in the early twentieth century. Someone had attempted to build high-end hotel rooms, but they were never completed. The current owner of the building had purchased it for a song and decided to just use it for office space. The unfinished hotel rooms were converted into offices, and Dorm's offices covered the entire third floor.

I entered the director of nursing's office, introduced myself to the secretary, and waited. I was summoned by a large, friendly young woman and entered a small office.

At the table sat an elderly, professionally dressed woman—Robin, the director of nursing. A second attendant was Brittany, a very attractive black woman, who was slender, with long dark hair, and very well dressed. A third woman, probably the most senior in years but with a youthful smile, silver hair, and more casual dress, was Ramona. Finally, the woman who brought me in was probably the youngest, and her name was Paige. The interview lasted about forty-five minutes. The questions were all appropriate, and I readily responded.

One question I found interesting was, "How do you keep yourself organized?"

Quickly, I pulled out my appointment book. "This is how I do it."

They all smiled, and Robin said, "Good answer!"

At the end of the interview, they thanked me for coming. Robin shook my hand. "We'll call in a few days with our decision."

When Paige called, she told them they had decided on another applicant. I was saddened, of course, but thought maybe it was meant to be.

Funny thing—a month later, Paige called again to ask if I was still interested. "We have another opening."

CHAPTER 19 FAMILY TROUBLES

I quickly responded yes.

This time, I met only with Brittany—a very informal meeting about the job requirements. We decided on a start date after my two-week notice at my current job.

I left feeling excited but a bit melancholy.

Back home, I typed my resignation for Regency Care. I had been there four years, and it was one of my best all-inclusive learning experiences in the medical field. I did bedside nursing; collaborated with patients from infants to seniors; worked in the home, hospital, nursing home, and alcohol rehab center; instructed aides and nurses; and supervised, developed orders for home care, coordinated teams, and put in a little human resource time. The job had been a great learning experience and allowed me to meet terrific people.

But I needed to move on to have more family time.

When I handed Amy my resignation, I had tears in my eyes. Amy teared up as well. She read the letter. "We will really miss you, but I wish you the best." Amy was insightful and knew the frustration all four of us supervisors felt.

Amanda asked, "Is there anything we can do to make you stay?"

"No, the schedule here doesn't give me enough time with my children. And my parents need more help, too. This new position will give me that time."

Amanda knew she could not guarantee that I would have more time with my family if I stayed with the company.

I sat down with Monica, Caleb, and Lewis and told them I was leaving. I had to force back the tears. Monica was first to give me a big hug and Caleb and Lewis followed. They all asked for details about the job and gave me good wishes.

Next, I needed to talk to the coordinators—Angela, Dana, and Peggy. By the time I was done, I felt as if someone had sapped all of my energy. I felt like a jelly roll.

Nursing, Yes I Do!

Those last two weeks flew by, as I had to ensure all my scheduled orders for services and home care visits were completed. Finally, that dreaded last day arrived. Everyone in the office was in the coordinators' section and they all got a hug. I just could not speak. I just waved, left, and cried all the way home.

Chapter 20

ANOTHER NEW BEGINNING

I had the weekend to recover from my farewells, and on Monday, I arrived at Dorm for my orientation meeting with Brittany. She took me around to meet the staff.

Each of the three supervisors—Brittany, Paige, and Ramona—had a team of assessor nurses. Three caseworker supervisors were each responsible for a team of caseworkers. Each case was assigned to a caseworker and a nurse to manage the services. They all appeared to be very happy and relaxed.

Tony was the assistant deputy of the social services program, and while he had an important title, he was a very down-to-earth and genuine man. Maureen was the case worker supervisor who worked alongside Brittany and oversaw the caseworkers in our team. She was just as warm and welcoming as Brittany. I met our team members last.

As soon as I saw Callie, we hugged each other. Great news! Callie was on Brittany's team, so we would be working together again.

As I strolled to my assigned desk, I noticed a caseworker sitting at a desk near Callie who was leaning back in his chair, talking on the phone with his feet on the desk. He hadn't been there during the introductions. After a couple of minutes, he hung up and stood so he could be introduced as well. He was a tall, very thin, pale man of about fifty years old who talked incessantly. He shook my hand. "Hi, I'm Peter, and I'll be working with you on some cases."

"Nice to meet you."

The other caseworker I would work with was Liam. He was a white-haired, boxy-built man who was about sixty years old, friendly, and well-versed in county rules and regulations. He had originally planned to get into sales but, for whatever reason, took his civil service exam and started his work there.

Brittany took me back to her office and gave me some pointers on working with county employees. "Our job is through a contract with the county, so we are somewhat of a guest consultant. Therefore, we must remember"—she leaned forward— "the county workers are in charge." She sat back again, smiling. "Most of the county workers are very compatible, but some have a pious attitude. You will find out quickly who those folks are. Basically . . . know that your place in this system is offering your medical expertise to determine medical appropriateness for home care."

"I understand."

She slid a black book across the desk to me. "Your Medicaid bible. Review as needed."

It was huge. I saw that first and foremost, I would have to familiarize myself with Medicaid and its provisions. This was something I knew very little about. Before I had started in-home care, I even got Medicare and Medicaid confused. At least I knew the differences by the time I started at Dorm, as that would have been embarrassing.

"The caseworkers are primarily responsible to know the regulations, but at times we have to write letters to a client or their representative if we find ourselves in a dispute about care services." At times, we would also have to appear for a fair hearing and argue our point to an appellant law judge.

Brittany also educated me on the contract company we worked for. The name was Cooperative Care, and while we had very little responsibility to them, on occasion, we would have to complete some volunteer work for

CHAPTER 20 ANOTHER NEW BEGINNING

them, as they were a nonprofit agency that not only employed us but did work for the community. They had their own administrative staff separate from the county, with offices on the fourth floor.

Brittany took me to meet their staff. Their offices were much nicer than ours. The staff was cordial and very professional. I was told they were planning a wine and cheese party for contributors and would seek our help for the event. Sounded nice. I could manage that.

I spent the first three days just reviewing regulations and going over paperwork. On the fourth day, I accompanied Callie and Liam on a community visit to see how such visits were done. We saw three clients.

Callie made a point of telling me, "I know it may be hard to do, but remember, this is 'hands-off' nursing. If a client asks us to do something medical, you must gracefully decline and offer to contact someone who can do it."

On Monday I met with Brittany, who said, "You are fine to take on your caseload independently."

That was exciting news I shared with Callie and the rest of the team. Callie replied, "You got your wings in one week! That's a record."

I was eager to begin. Since the caseworkers had all the last appointments, I depended on them to tell me when visits were due. Soon I felt comfortable reminding the caseworker of upcoming visits, the micromanager that I am.

We made joint appointments with most of the visits, but at times, we would go solo. I must admit, it felt weird not to do any hands-on nursing. Our visits generally went as follows.

The caseworker started by asking about the aide or nursing services in general, questions like, are they on time, respectful, and doing the tasks; are there any environmental issues we should know about like the heat, water, or neighborhood, etc. My part would involve looking at their prescription bottles, confirming their pharmacy, physicians, changes in health status, and current functional status. I would ensure that the care plan for the nurse or aide met the client's needs. If the client were hospitalized, and possibly placed in the rehabilitation center, we would evaluate them there to assess the need for any changes. If so, the caseworker would have to revisit the house before they went home to ensure the electricity, water, etc., still worked. A family member would meet the caseworker to let him or her check the house.

We usually made our visits in the afternoon, and my mornings were generally spent completing paperwork from the visits the day before. I would hand my paperwork to Brittany for review. If there were corrections, she would return it with a note on it. Her notes gradually decreased.

Our days were easy, and we were always having potluck lunches. I found myself making soups, chicken, salads, and stromboli for the office. We used the old ballrooms for special lunches and events. The three ballrooms had tall, tiled ceilings, rich dark woodwork, and five- to six-foot-high fireplaces reminiscent of the 1920s. The rooms all had pocket doors that connected to other portions of the ballroom. You could almost hear the music from a long-ago era and smell the tobacco that filled the room back in the day.

A great deli across the street from our building sold excellent food from breakfast to lunch. The name was Gino's, and it was really convenient for lunches. The owner was originally from Brooklyn, and a sign at the register said We Do Not Sell Pop, We Sell Soda.

Precarious Situations

Most of our home calls were not in the best neighborhoods. Once I met Peter at a case and, as I pulled up on the street a few cars behind him, a young, poorly dressed woman banged on my door. "Do you have the stuff?"

CHAPTER 20 ANOTHER NEW BEGINNING

Peter hollered, "That girl is a county worker, and she works with me."

At that, the woman turned and walked away. I thanked Peter for that.

For most cases, the services we approved were appropriate, but at times the client was really taking Medicaid for a ride.

I got so tired of hearing clients say, "I pay for this, and I am entitled to this care."

I would bite my tongue and hold back my comments. But I was thinking, *No, all the taxpayers are paying for this, and I'm here to make sure you have your services.*

A classic example of how county funds were being misused involved a young man I'll call Mr. Dunbar. He had been shot by a companion in a drug deal and was now paralyzed from the waist down. Even though he had a criminal record, he was a victim in this matter.

Considering his permanent disability, the county paid an exorbitant amount of money to ensure his home was safe and accessible. This involved exterior and interior work and appliances. Several weeks after the remodeling and appliance installation, Mr. Dunbar made a claim that appliances and various home décor items had been stolen. There was concern that the patient had planned the burglary, but that could not be proven.

Dorm services were meant to supplement care by family and friends in the home, but in this case, we ended up providing twenty-four hours of care per day, including a few hours of nursing because of medications, with the remaining time being personal care aide services.

Our semiannual visits with Mr. Dunbar were always entertaining. He was a master of confabulation, manipulation, and arrogance. Once, he called to tell me his aide would not go to the laundromat at midnight like he requested. We already suspected he was still carrying on drug deals in the home but could not prove it. The aides and nurses either did not see the activity or were afraid to say anything.

I asked, "Why do you send your aide out at midnight to do the laundry when this should be done during daylight hours, as on the care plan?"

He growled, "I need her here during the day, and she can do that while I sleep."

I wondered what he had in that laundry basket besides laundry for the aide to deliver on his behalf.

I continued to push the issue of safety for the staff and asked him to consider an earlier time. "You can be left alone for a couple of hours. You're able to use the phone."

He agreed to this but did not follow through.

I spoke to the caseworker supervisor, Maureen, about decreasing his hours from twenty-four to sixteen hours per day in light of the abuse of services, and she agreed.

We submitted the request to the administrative office, and they notified Mr. Dunbar. He filed a grievance, which resulted in continued twenty-four care until a fair hearing would be held.

Over the next three years, a fair hearing notice was sent to Mr. Dunbar twice, however each time, he requested the hearing to be rescheduled.

Our staff occasionally served clients who had run-ins with the law. I once made a home call to a patient and listened to her woes about her son, whom she admitted was on the loose, wrongly accused of shooting a police officer. I was probably in the house for about an hour.

The next day, I read in the paper that police had located a man hiding in his mother's closet—at the same address I had visited the day before—and identified him as the man who had shot a police officer. I got chills.

One of my co-workers told me she had been at a house and was introduced to a man they called a family friend, but she remembered the face

CHAPTER 20 ANOTHER NEW BEGINNING

as a man who had been on the news as a suspect in a series of burglaries. A few days later, the police caught up with him.

Dealing with Some Troublesome Caseworkers

Patients weren't the only ones who could act dubiously when it came to applying the rules. Occasionally, I was asked to help another team if they were busy. Once a caseworker approached me to see one of her cases because her nurse had been out sick for a while. Visits were supposed to be done every six months, and this one had not been done for a year.

She handed me the forms from the previous visit. "See the patient and complete two sets. Date one for six months ago and one with your current visit—anyway, you know the drill."

My mouth dropped open. I thought, *No, I do not.*

I saw the client and entered the date that I saw her.

I handed the documents to Paige, the nursing supervisor for that team. I said, "This case was late as per the caseworker," and left it at that.

I was getting ready for my first vacation since starting the new job, and on the day before my vacation, Liam and I visited one of our senior ladies at the rehabilitation center. We had to ensure she was still appropriate for home care and develop her new care plan. She was stable and ready to go home in two days. Liam had to call her son to see the house before she went home to make sure all the utilities were on.

I was already aware of Liam's lackadaisical attitude to things, and it was midwinter, so I reminded him, "Please do not forget to call the son and visit the home."

When I returned from vacation, I had messages from the home care agency—there was no running water. I looked at Liam and asked if he had visited the house to check the utilities.

He laughed. "No, why?"

"They had no water to give her a bath, so the agency had to provide water in jugs."

He laughed again. "They could have melted some of the snow."

I gaped. "Seriously?"

Liam was not the only lackadaisical one. Peter would do as little work as possible and gloat about it. I happened to look at some of the messages from the home care agency to Peter. One mentioned a shooting at the home across the street from one of our cases. The memo was dated two months earlier. I showed it to him.

He just snickered. "I never read those messages."

I was aggravated because it is just inconsiderate to jeopardize someone's safety like that. I immediately went to Maureen with the memo.

She called Peter into the office. Maureen was a very kind and delicate lady, and in her usual softhearted manner, she told Peter he needed to pay better attention to those messages.

One bad habit the caseworkers had was not returning calls to clients or agency staff who left voicemails in a timely manner.

The caseworkers were supposed to manage cases, and every so often, a pious caseworker would remind us of this. Home care had to be authorized by a physician, and sometimes, we might have to contact the doctor because of a change in a patient's medical condition. Some caseworkers felt it was their role to do this. I would explain why it might be a better idea to have the nurse call the doctor. Most agreed with this, but I might rarely get a response like, "Who do you think you are?"

I would respond by saying, "The nurse."

Christmas at Dorm

As at any company, not all work in patient care is directly work-related. Christmas, for example, has a way of melting people's hearts and encouraging

CHAPTER 20 ANOTHER NEW BEGINNING

them to work together for the benefit of co-workers. Ninety-eight percent of the staff participated in a joint Christmas party for Cooperative Care and the Dorm program at the end of 2002. Callie was on the committee and pulled me in as well.

Liam played Santa and placed the names of those willing to participate in a gift exchange in a hat. After he had all the names, he pulled from the hat the name of a co-worker we each should purchase a five- to ten-dollar gift for.

Sandy from administration loved homemade baked goods, so she brought around a list for people to donate a fresh baked dessert. *No store-bought baked goods allowed* was the motto on the list. I signed up to bring a spice cake.

Someone from Cooperative Care arranged for food delivery and collected a nominal amount from each person for the food and beverages. It was for lunch, but the food was like having dinner, as the menu included rigatoni, roast beef sandwiches, green salad, and pasta salad.

The plan was to use one of the old ballrooms. As I mentioned before, our offices were in a repurposed dance hall and intended hotel, but the ballrooms had been left unattended and were a bit of a mess. About twelve of us cleaned as best we could. We polished the woodwork and swept and mopped the floors. By the time we were done, the room smelled of lemon and pine.

I was also on the decoration committee. We brought down the Christmas tree from the administration office, along with a large chair covered with a fluffy red blanket for Santa. For a week before the party, we met daily at lunch to make centerpieces. I worked harder getting ready for this party than for my regular job!

We had a fundraising raffle as well, and it was filled primarily with handmade items like blankets, scarves, socks, and paintings. I had no idea that the staff I worked with was so talented!

Nursing, Yes I Do!

Sandra was one of the nurses who was an amazing painter and wrote short stories. She usually painted on shale but would tinker with other things. I bought two of her winter scene shale pieces, and when I saw the nature painting on a saw that she put in the raffle, I had to have it for Ethan. I decided that if I did not win it, I would ask her to paint me another one.

The day arrived, and those of us on the decoration committee went down to the room about ten o'clock in the morning to set up the centerpieces. Sandy came down and set out the deserts on the long table. There was no shortage of baked goods. We all gave her a hand.

The tables and chairs Cooperative Care had rented had been delivered and set up with white tablecloths. By noon all the staff arrived, with two hours for lunch that day.

The raffle table was set up on one side of the room. The money collected would go toward the party for the next year. I could not wait to place tickets in the cup for Sandra's painted saw.

I had not met the CEO of Cooperative Care before then. He wanted to say a few words before lunch to thank everyone for their cooperation and to wish us all a Merry Christmas and Happy New Year. He called up Tony, who said a few words about the great teamwork between the county workers and Cooperative Care and ended with heartfelt wishes for happy holidays.

We eagerly started the table calls to get our lunch and desserts. After about an hour, we set up Santa. Since the gifts were already under the tree, he called the names on the list, and his trusty elves—me included—passed out the gifts. Since Liam had a bit of a sense of humor, it was quite entertaining.

After that, the raffle winners were drawn. As they held up the bag of tickets for Sandra's painted saw, I held my breath and . . . I won! It would be a special present for my hubby, since he was so handy around the house.

CHAPTER 20 ANOTHER NEW BEGINNING

Before we knew it, the time was over, and fortunately, we had a few other volunteers to help with cleanup. Whew, who could work after all that? That afternoon we weren't very productive.

Other Events with Cooperative Care

The next work-related social event was a wine and cheese party for all the company's contributors. It was to be held in the ballroom labeled as the Paris Ballroom on the mezzanine. This was a different room than the one we used for Christmas, but it was in a similar state. Therefore, we had a full day of cleaning to do.

Since we had already gone through this with the Christmas party, we knew what to do. Two days before the event, we all came in wearing our old clothes. We brought in pails, rags, mops, and cleaning solutions. After six hours with twelve of us working, the room eventually smelled and looked as clean as we could get it.

The event was scheduled to start at six o'clock on Friday evening. Those of us who were helping to prepare for the evening dressed in semi-formal attire and were assigned to serve the wine and appetizers. At this event, I learned how to use a corkscrew to open a bottle of wine.

We worked hand-in-hand with the staff from Cooperative Care and got to know them a little better. I developed a fondness for the girls who were responsible for the marketing, event planning, and outreach, but I was not too sure about the CEO, Frank. Something about him made me leery. Maybe it was the lack of eye contact when he spoke to me or the loose handshake, but I felt something was not right with him. But I did enjoy meeting the rich folk who contributed to Cooperative Care.

Personal Life Changes

I was so grateful for the time off I had with this job. It allowed me to be around my children more, spend time with my husband, and take care

263

Nursing, Yes I Do!

of my parents as they aged. My dad was really declining; medical reports indicated that he had metastatic cancer.

For about a year, I had almost every Friday off, so I took my dad and mom to doctors' appointments.

Chapter 21

FAIR HEARINGS

Despite their name, patient hearings were often far from fair.

My first experience with one involved an eight-year-old boy with total care needs involving feeding, hygiene, toileting, and mobility. He had a feeding tube for nutrition, diapers for bladder and bowel excretions, and a specialized wheelchair for mobility. He was nonverbal and communicated with vocal noises or facial expressions. He had a seizure disorder and minimal purposeful movement of his limbs.

The child lived with his parents, and while they had both been trained to take care of the child by hospital staff, they resisted responsibility. Therefore, for eight years, private duty nursing had been supplied for twenty hours per day. The only time the parents took responsibility for the child was from 2 p.m. to 6 p.m., and he slept during that time.

Once, the child had a seizure during that time, and the mother called the doctor's office in a panic, not knowing what to do. She was told how to handle the child until the seizure stopped.

The father had a maintenance job and worked forty hours per week, Monday through Friday. Mom did not work, but ensured there was food and supplies for the child, while caring for one other child who was well and approaching age five.

At this point I considered asking for a decrease in the hours of the private duty nurse, since when the five-year-old started school, Mom would

Nursing, Yes I Do!

have more time to care for her ill son. I brought this up with the assigned caseworker, Liam.

He laughed. "It'll never work."

"I'm only considering a decrease to seventeen hours as opposed to twenty."

He just shook his head.

When we went to make the home call, I brought it up to mom. She immediately turned me down.

I didn't give in. "I'm proposing the following schedule for the nurse—11 p.m to 8 a.m., then 11 a.m. to 7 p.m."

She adamantly refused, even though I reminded her the open times were during periods when no treatments or medications were due. "You can just have good bonding time with your son."

We left without her agreeing, but I convinced Liam to put in for the decrease.

Whenever the client or representative refuses a decrease in service, you have to maintain the current schedule in the interim of a fair hearing.

Just before our next scheduled visit, we attended the fair hearing. My role was to report the nursing needs. I drew up an estimated timeline of the time necessary for each task, excluding monitoring the child. The total time on tasks per day was six hours.

Liam and I represented Dorm, and the family brought one of the nurses, as well as a friend who claimed to be studying law. The nurses are not supposed to appear as witnesses because as employees of the agency that had the contract with Dorm, there would be a conflict of interest. This nurse stated that she no longer worked for the agency and was now a friend of the family.

The hearing officer was efficient and listened to all that was said. His closing comments were favorable to the family, so we could not decrease the time.

CHAPTER 21 FAIR HEARINGS

Liam said, "I told you so."

"Well, we tried."

This was truly a learning experience, and my next fair hearing involved an adult who lived in a nursing home and wanted to go home with Dorm services. This was another case with Liam, and I was determined to win this case based on what I saw.

The client was a sixty-three-year-old male, weighing 300 pounds, non-ambulatory due to paralysis of his legs after a stroke, with weakness in both arms. He could use an electric wheelchair within the facility, but the apartment he planned to move into would not be accessible because the halls were too narrow for the wheelchair.

He had no family or friend support and would need an aide to assist with feeding, bathing, open medication dressing, toileting, mechanical transfer, shopping, doctor appointments, errands, and paying bills.

Because of the disability in his arms, he could not even call for help by phone, although a Personal Emergency Response System button could be installed. With this in mind, he could be left only for one-hour intervals since he needed repositioning every two hours to prevent pressure sores.

After I spoke with the discharge planner and the doctor, we agreed that unless his home environment could accommodate all of his needs that were currently met in the nursing home, he was best left in his current environment.

I asked the discharge planner to please have the physician write that on the order sheet, and she did so. This was beneficial to our program and to maintain his safety.

The Fair Hearing was set for two months later, and I had the doctor's note stating that the patient's care needs mirrored what he already had in the nursing home.

Nursing, Yes I Do!

I attended the meeting with Liam and our medical director. The client was there, with no family or friend support.

After presenting all the information, the hearing officer said, "The client's needs are best met at the nursing home."

The client was irate and insisted on appealing this decision.

"You certainly have that right," the officer said, "but in the interim, you'll remain in the nursing home."

As we walked out to the parking lot, Liam said, "Congratulations. I'm really impressed with your work on this."

"Thank you," I said. "It was a commonsense matter."

I was shocked by some of the cases we served, in which patients were already receiving home care.

One example was a woman in her fifties with progressive multiple sclerosis as well as being labeled as moderately mentally impaired. Our program authorized sixteen hours per day of aide service, from 8 a.m. to midnight. She was only alone during her sleeping hours. This lady was nonverbal, non-ambulatory, and needed help in all daily living activities. At the time her case was initiated, she had some movement in her arms and legs and could push the emergency response button on her wrist. As the years passed, all her limbs became weaker.

On my visit to assess her needs, I asked her to try to push the button.

She couldn't.

When Peter and I left the house, I voiced concern for her safety. "To avoid twenty-four-hour care, placement is the best option."

He responded, "We should just leave well enough alone."

"Seriously?"

On my return to the office, I spoke to Brittany, who agreed with me. She immediately called a meeting with Peter and his supervisor, Maureen.

CHAPTER 21 FAIR HEARINGS

Maureen also agreed and told Peter to call Adult Protective Services and the Office for the Developmentally Disabled. "Arrange for a meeting at the client's home with you and Aubrey."

Considering the urgency, the meeting was held the next day. Three people arrived: two from the ODD and one from APS.

We all sat down and started out with a delightful conversation about the upcoming Christmas holiday. I waited for a good segue, and then brought up the topic of the client's inability to press the emergency call button. I depended on the representatives from the ODD to help with this.

They listened intently to my report on the patient's case. They said Peter had given them a different picture.

I was not surprised. Those caseworkers had no sense of urgency.

I knew asking the patient to press the button on her wrist would upset her, but I asked anyway.

As I expected, we all watched the client try and try again to push that button over a five-minute period. Finally, tears rolled down her face.

The reps from ODD became very sympathetic, offering her soothing comments. One of them asked, "Could you increase her hours?"

Before Peter could open his mouth, I said, "You know she needs twenty-four hour care, and we cannot do that. It is in the best interest of the client to have her transported to County Hospital in the interim of placement. That way physicians can properly medically assess her before she's placed."

They all nodded—except Peter. I'm sure I was stepping on his toes, but he really did not know how to manage such situations.

Another case involved a darling little twelve-year-old boy with encephalitis. I'll call him Devin. This condition was the result of a high fever he'd had when he was four years old and left him in a vegetative state. For the

Nursing, Yes I Do!

first two years, his mom, Blair, provided the bulk of the care, even though she worked full-time as a pharmacist at a local hospital.

Our program initially provided nurses for her from 8 a.m. to 6 p.m. Blair arrived home at 4:30 p.m., and the ninety-minute overlap before the nurse left let her have her own dinner and help the nurse during Devin's bath time.

On the weekends, the nurse was there from 8 a.m. to 4 p.m., which allowed Blair to run errands and visit family and friends.

When the child turned nine years old, Blair developed a relationship with a man who lived nearby. She asked for extra hours to allow her to pursue this relationship. The hours were increased to eighteen hours per day. Before long, Blair was living with this man most of the time, and the hours were increased to twenty-four hours per day.

Blair came over frequently during the day to make sure supplies were in the house, but eventually, even this seemed to change. She demanded more of the nurses. She wanted the nurses to lift her son in a cradle wrap because this was how she did it; however, it is not the recommended way for the nurses to use proper body mechanics. The cradle wrap lift—wrapping the patient and picking them up—does not support the patient as well as a mechanical lift and puts too much strain on the nurse's back.

The nurses noticed that the heat in the house during the winter was not high enough. They had to really bundle up the child and themselves to stay warm. If a nurse issued a concern to Blair about the heat, she became vengeful to the nurse and made it even more unpleasant for the nurse. Blair also left their family dog in the house for the nurses to care for.

After a while, staffing the case became more and more difficult because the word was out about this difficult mother. New nurses refused to go, and existing nurses wanted off the case.

CHAPTER 21 FAIR HEARINGS

All of these issues were reported to me when I was assigned to the case as the assessor nurse. I discussed the aforementioned issues with Devin's mom, and she just laughed.

I remained firm. "If we continue to have less and less staff to serve your son, we'll have no choice but to recommend placement."

Blair fired back, "Just try it!" She glowered. "Staff the case and mind your own business."

She was obviously dealing with a lot of mixed emotions about her son and the relationship with her male friend. I wondered if this man was giving her a problem about her son. "I recommend that you and I have a meeting, along with the caseworkers and agency representative. Your boyfriend can come, too, if you want."

"No."

I brought this information back to Robin, Brittany, Maureen, and Liam. They agreed a meeting should be scheduled.

Robin took the case file. "Since she said no to you. I'll call Blair myself and advise her of the importance of this meeting."

The meeting was scheduled for three days later. Liam, Maureen, Brittany, and I sat down to draft a list of issues to discuss.

Because the case was a twenty-four-hour pediatric matter, we had quite a large crowd: the director of nursing and the supervisor from the staffing agency attended, as well as Robin, Brittany, Maureen, Liam, and I. We gathered around a conference table in our office.

Blair showed up, but her boyfriend did not.

Robin tried to start the meeting with our list of concerns, but Blair immediately began issuing complaints about negligent nursing staff not following her instructions. "And I get no communication or help from Dorm."

Brittany pulled out a paper and pen. "Please give us specifics, so we can take corrective action."

Blair yelled, "I do not want Dorm to make out care plans for the nurses—I will. I do not want nurses who question how to reach me, question the temperature of my house, or refuse to take care of the dog. The dog is my son's pet, and that makes him an extension of the care for my son."

Brittany dutifully wrote all this down.

I really had to contain myself and not roll my eyes.

"Let's take each issue one at a time." Robin clicked her own pen and slid Brittany's list in front of herself and started with care plans. These are made out by our staff in collaboration with the doctor's orders and in compliance with the state department of health. If you disagree, you are free to private pay for your own staff."

Mom didn't reply.

Robin checked off care plans and moved to the next item on the list, contact information. "The nurses need to know how to reach you in case of an emergency, whether it is related to your son or the house."

Blair folded her arms and looked away.

Robin made another check. "The temperature of the house needs to be comfortable for your son." She cocked her head. "I'm told the temperature in the house is so low that your son's fingers were ice-cold despite being under two heavy blankets."

When Blair still didn't reply, Robin checked that off, too.

"The dog, as with any pet, is not the responsibility of the nurse." Robin put her pen down and leaned forward. "I'm sure that out of compassion, many of the nurses have helped take care of the dog and allowed it some bonding time with your son, but it is out of the realm of health care. We cannot expect the nurses to take on that responsibility." She leaned back and picked up her pen again. "Please note while pet therapy is used in

CHAPTER 21 FAIR HEARINGS

residential facilities, they have separate staff members to take care of the pets and the therapy time. Perhaps you can keep the dog with *you* and speak to the doctor about pet therapy."

Blair raised her eyebrows. "Well, *perhaps* it is time for me to get an attorney."

Maureen piped in. "That's your right, and we would be happy to discuss it further with them." In the interim, we really need to discuss the staffing problem."

The director of nursing from the staffing agency spoke up. "I have only three nurses who are willing to fill these shifts. When I have no staff nurse to fill the shift, I must send one of my supervisors. I cannot keep using my supervisors to fill shifts, especially the overnight shifts, as that puts them in a dangerous position—working a twenty-four-hour day."

The meeting lasted an hour, and in the end, we decided to contract a second agency to help with the staffing. Blair agreed to that plan.

Brittany and Maureen called Liam and me into a meeting.

"You remember Mr. Dunbar," Maureen said.

I sure did. He was the one who'd been shot in a drug deal gone wrong. We'd made three unsuccessful attempts to schedule a fair hearing with him.

"There was a shooting in his home . . ." Maureen hesitated. "While one of the nurses was there."

"What?" My heart felt as if it had stopped. "Is she okay?"

"Yes, the nurse is fine," Brittany said.

I grabbed a chair and sat down. "What happened?"

Brittany and Maureen took turns telling Liam and me the story. "Apparently a drug deal had been going on in the home, and it ended badly, with a male visitor shot. He was rushed to the hospital with life-threatening injuries."

"What about Mr. Dunbar?" Liam asked.

"He was transferred to the hospital as well," Maureen said. "The police did that because they did not feel it was a safe environment."

I thanked God for that—and that our nurse escaped all right.

After a week, Mr. Dunbar was transferred to the county home, despite his multiple attempts to be transferred home.

Our prayers we answered, as we never had to provide him with home care services again.

Imprisoned by Snow

Working in the heart of the city came with some disadvantages when bad weather hit. For some reason, it was a hub for higher wind gusts. Some of the buildings had a rope around them for pedestrians to hold onto at those times.

An ice storm hit the second winter I worked there. After an early home call, I returned to the office and parked on the street closer to the building. But every time I tried to open the car door; the wind blew it closed again. It took three attempts and fifteen minutes before I successfully got out of the car. And that was not the end of it.

As I walked toward the building, I struggled to prevent myself from slipping on the ice. I wound up grabbing light posts as the gusts increased. When I finally made it into the building, I was a sweaty mess, covered with ice.

If that were not enough, we were hit by a major snowstorm a month later, the week of Thanksgiving. By 10:30 a.m. Monday, the powers-that-be decided to send us home. The elevators were turned off, so we had to take the stairs. As we reached the parking lot across the street from the building, we decided to make sure everyone's car could start and could get out of the parking lot. Two cars needed to be pushed out.

CHAPTER 21 FAIR HEARINGS

By the time I was on my way home, it was 12:30 p.m., and the city streets were gridlocked. The temperature outside was fifteen degrees, and with the wind blowing snow around, it was hard to see anything.

I had my cell phone, so I called Ethan. "I'm headed home, but there's no guarantee when I'll get there."

Hours ticked by: 1:30 p.m. turned into 2:30 p.m. and then 3:30 p.m. and then 4:30 p.m., and I had only moved one block.

Within the next thirty minutes, there was finally some movement. Police officers guided us to enter a parking ramp. I got out of the car and followed the others and was directed into the county sheriff's holding center. Well, this was a first, as I never had the pleasure of being in jail.

A tall muscular officer led us to a hall with plenty of uncomfortable chairs. Another officer asked us if we would like a cup of coffee, and all twelve of us said yes.

My first instinct was to call the hotel across the street for a room. They had no vacancy. "I'm sorry," the clerk said, "But we have several school buses of children staying here."

My heart sank. I was not going to sleep in a jail cell. And the coffee tasted like sludge.

I went back to the hall, where officers were passing out dinner in boxes. Ugh, prisoner food. I suppose I should be grateful I was out of the cold . . . but a jail!

After a few minutes, I was in a deep conversation with the woman next to me. That was a great distraction. Her name was Zoe and she mentioned that she was ill and needed medication, which was at home. Her boyfriend was bringing it to her. She handed me a folded paper and followed with, "Please do not open this unless I collapse. It is my medical history." I prayed I would not have to.

Nursing, Yes I Do!

Zoe did not want to stay at the jail either, so we decided to walk across the street to the hotel and sleep in chairs or on the floor if we had to. We stood up and headed for the door.

That lovely tall muscular officer stood in front of us with his hands on his hips. "Where are you going?"

"Thank you for your hospitality," I said, "but we are meeting her boyfriend with her medication across the street."

He could not argue with that.

Zoe had no boots on, so I held her up as we went through the snow. When we arrived, I asked desperately at the front desk if they had any rooms or blankets available. They had neither.

We headed to the restaurant/bar. The room was packed. People were lined up four deep at the bar, ordering drinks and watching the hockey game on TV.

Zoe was getting pale and tired. I took her arm. "Let's find some seats."

A couple at a nearby table noticed how ill Zoe looked and invited us to sit with them.

We introduced ourselves and learned they weren't actually a couple—they had just met. The woman, Gina, was also a nurse, and the guy was a school bus driver. We shared stories of how we had ended up there.

Soon Zoe's boyfriend arrived. "We might be able to at least get into a storage room for the night if the staff sees how sick you are." He helped her up, and they left.

After another hour, the school bus driver left as well, to check on his students. Gina and I searched the other public rooms to locate a couple of comfy chairs to sleep in. We found two high-back wing chairs and dragged them into the main hall outside a ballroom.

"My car is right out front," she said, "and I have blankets in there. I'll bring them in."

CHAPTER 21 FAIR HEARINGS

While she was gone, I placed my jacket on the other chair to show anyone walking by that it was taken.

Gina returned with a pillow and two blankets. "I'm sorry I only have one pillow."

"Did you not know you would need two pillows today?"

She laughed. We were surrounded by a few more chairs and some tables. The man on our right was a chain smoker, but neither one of us dared to ask him to stop. Tension levels were up all over, so we just dealt with it.

I am not sure who fell asleep first. We exhausted ourselves talking, until a sudden silence... the next thing I knew, I woke up with a horrible taste in my mouth and a blasting headache. I twisted around in the chair, trying to get comfortable.

Gina woke up. "What is that horrible smell?"

"Stale smoke and booze." I looked around and saw multiple male bodies lying on the floor. They reeked of alcohol.

There was a definite hustle of people in the lobby, so we headed that way. As we peaked out the window, we saw men in orange jumpsuits and parkas shoveling the road. People were milling around outside, helping each other get their cars shoveled out.

After about an hour, there was actual movement of cars on the road as well as the City Crossway expressway.

Gina and I said farewell and headed to our cars and then homeward.

Chapter 22

SUPERVISORY CHANGES

When I had started at Dorm, the three nursing supervisors were Ramona, Paige, and Brittany. Two years in, Ramona had retired, and we gave her a glorious send-off dinner at the Old Orchard Inn. I was sad to see her go, because she was so down to earth and a real pleasure to work with.

With this retirement, a nurse from the waivered program team was promoted to the supervisor program. That left an opening for a nurse in the waivered program, so I decided to apply. This team was composed of three registered nurses and three caseworkers. The caseload involved clients with higher needs, so these workers had more advanced training than the staff I had worked with and welcomed the added experience. I was offered and accepted the position.

I was warned about a few of the team members' personalities but was happy to hear that with the recent shuffling of supervisors, Brittany was also moved to that team, and I was so grateful.

The billing system for this team was also a bit different. Brittany gave me a book with the team's policies and procedures. "You won't be assigned any cases for about one week."

In that time, I would review the book and shadow a nurse. The job entailed obtaining the medical orders for all Dorm patients, intake for new clients, home calls only for pediatric nursing cases, and signing off on approval for Medicaid nursing home cases.

CHAPTER 22 SUPERVISORY CHANGES

The other nurses on the team were Candy and Marianne. I had spent time with them in the lunchroom at times and felt very comfortable with them. Candy was a fair-skinned, fair-haired gal with a very calm disposition . . . sometimes too calm. Marianne had a light olive complexion with dark hair and presented herself as a bit sharp-tongued—bossy yet hysterical when she told stories.

The first week, I shadowed Marianne since she had seniority. I was told it was best to not cross her, or you might be tossed into an abyss never to be heard of again. I nodded a lot to avoid saying the wrong thing.

Since intake was the start of the process, we started with that. All cases started with a phone call with a request for care and a description of the needs. Joan was our intake person, and she was a kind, soft-spoken, motherly gal. She got the call first, gathered information, and then passed it on to the nurse.

I enjoyed this part, as the transcripts were always interesting. They came from various sources, including, but not limited to, doctor's offices, community outreach centers, hospitals, patient homes, etc. We took paper notes first and then transferred them to a computer database.

Filing cabinets held the new cases and existing cases awaiting medical orders, filed in the order of attempts to obtain orders. If someone really needed help at home, time was vital, so we had to call the physician.

Our new pediatric cases generally came with orders to start services as soon as possible. Updated doctor orders were required every six months for adult home care aide cases and every four months for pediatric nursing care cases. Two months before the due date, we sent a letter to the primary medical doctor with a follow-up thirty days later, if necessary. In most cases, the orders came back within the first month, which was ideal.

Community visits were only for the specialized pediatric cases on the waivered Medicaid program. My first shadowed visit with Marianne included Terry as well since she was the client's caseworker. Terry was very

Nursing, Yes I Do!

girl-next-door with fair skin, small features, blue eyes, and perfectly styled, curly hair. Her voice was soft, and her manner showed gentle kindness.

The patient was a five-year-old with encephalitis. He was nonverbal and nonmobile, with brain activity only allowing the vital centers to work, such as breathing and heart rate. We provided a nurse for respite for the family six hours per day and eight hours overnight. During our visit, the mother told us of a new treatment using in-home oxygen tents. The neurologist had completed a PET (positron emission tomography) scan of the brain.

She gave us a copy of the results and pointed to the areas of poor oxygenation, as explained by the neurologist. "He's confident the treatment will reverse the brain damage."

We all gave her our support.

In the meantime, I observed the child arching his back—an obvious type of seizure.

But the mother said, "Look, he is getting better already."

"That is great news." I forced a smile.

As in my prior role, these assessments were hands-off, so giving any opinion opposing the neurologist would not serve any purpose. Our role was to determine the nursing need and confirm whether it was appropriate under Medicaid guidelines. Marianne and Terry knew the guidelines well and explained the justification to me. They approved the services for another four months. I agreed that it seemed appropriate.

My next nursing case with Marianne was with one of Pat's cases. Pat was a stunningly attractive gal, and she flaunted it. She was tall and slender with an olive complexion and dark hair, and dressed in popular styles. She frequently primped her hair and makeup during the day, and in conversation, her opinions on style, food, houses, religion, and similar topics were the only ones that mattered.

CHAPTER 22 SUPERVISORY CHANGES

Pat strolled around the house like she had full power, until Marianne spoke up. That appeared to put Pat in her own little space. I think Pat was just trying to show off to the new person—me.

This was another patient with a seizure disorder, but this child was more mentally alert and mobile. We had approved a nurse for Monday through Friday from 3 p.m. to 6 p.m. During this time, the nurse would get the child off the bus, make sure he had a light snack, give him his Tegretol (a medication to prevent convulsions) and get him started on his homework. He was on a low dose of Tegretol four times per day, as that worked well for him. His mother got home between 5:30 and 6 p.m.

The family had just purchased a specially trained dog to sense the aura of a seizure coming on and signal the parents. The dog was a beautiful golden retriever that would assist the parents during the overnight, during playtime if they were not in the room, and eventually throughout the day, possibly eliminating the need for a nurse.

The company representative was coming to the house shortly after us, and as we were interested, we asked if we could stay to observe. The mother agreed.

When the representative for the company arrived, the mother told her there had been a recent problem with the dog. "He growls," she said, "and at one point, he snapped at me."

The representative nodded. "The dog needs to know he is not the leader of the pack." She gave the mom verbal and written instructions on how to handle the dog.

Follow-up reports from this mother indicated all was well with the dog.

The ability to approve nursing home cases required a day of training, which was provided by the state department of health. We were given a certificate that authorized us to review patient review instruments (PRI) and screens and determine the appropriateness of skilled nursing home care.

The woman who gave us our training was like a nurse out of the 1950s. Tall, broad-shouldered, and made up with dark red lipstick, she also had dyed, jet-black hair. She wore a lab coat over a long black skirt and a white blouse.

The most confusing part of the training had to do with determining if a patient had mental retardation or a mental illness, and then ensuring the services met their needs. Ongoing authorizations were done on these patients in compliance with the health department.

Once per week, each of us had to take a shift answering calls from clients in the community up to 5 p.m., to fulfill the policy of our program availability until that hour. This time was primarily for troubleshooting issues, and in most cases, care would be postponed until the next day.

One evening, Marianne was taking the calls, and since I was shadowing her, I listened to this conversation.

The client said, "Your caseworker only gave me an aide for Monday, Wednesday, and Friday. Today is Tuesday so I have no aide, and I'm hungry."

Marianne said, "Ma'am, do you live alone?"

"Yes."

"Is there a family member or friend we can call?"

"I have seven children," the client told her, "but we cannot call them."

"Do they all live out of town?"

"No, two live upstairs, and the others live here in the city."

Marianne looked at me and rolled her eyes. She said to the client, calmly, "Can you tell me why we cannot call any of them?"

"That is none of your business."

"I am sure the caseworker explained to you that our program only supplements what you and your family and friends can do."

CHAPTER 22 SUPERVISORY CHANGES

"I have no one to help me," the client whined.

"Are you saying you are not safe to live alone without help?"

"Yes, I need someone here all the time."

Marianne made a note of this. "Ma'am, I will have to call an ambulance to take you to the hospital, because you are telling me you are not safe right now."

"I do not need to go the hospital," the client snapped. "You need to send me an aide for eighteen hours a day."

"I am sorry, if you are saying you have eighteen hours per day of needs, you are not appropriate for home care." Marianne used a soft, placating tone. "Your needs will be best met in an adult home."

"I am not going to a nursing home!"

Marianne's voice turned firm. "All right, then I must go back to whether you have family or friends to assist you in addition to aide services. If not, you leave me no choice but to call 911 for your safety."

"Don't you dare call 911. I am not unsafe."

"It is now 5 p.m., when did you last eat?"

"I had meatloaf an hour ago." She slammed the phone down.

Marianne placed her phone on the hook and looked at me. We exchanged exasperated eye rolls.

Upheaval

News broke out of severe monetary issues with Cooperative Care, and it was all over the local news. How embarrassing for all of us.

Board members of Cooperative Care and administrators from Dorm had meetings and more meetings. When the dust finally settled, the nurses received notice that Dorm would find another agency to function as our contracting company. I never did learn why the county couldn't just hire us.

In the interim, we could work as an independent contractor, however, each of us had to hold our own malpractice insurance with at least one million dollars of coverage and to add Dorm as a covered party as well. Since most of us did not have malpractice insurance, we had to apply for it. Fortunately, it was not too expensive, but it was still not something any of us had budgeted for.

Brittany sought out a new partner organization, and the Multicultural Community Center agreed to take us on. The transition went smoothly, although our contract with the MCC was very different from the one we had with Cooperative Care. There was no need to help with fundraising, as MCC was pretty well set with volunteers. Alternate arrangements were made for donations.

And The Beat Goes On

I enjoyed my new position on the waivered program team, as it was more challenging than my earlier position. My day started with one of the rotating tasks between Candy, Marianne, and me. Usually, after a couple of hours, we would take a break and tell stories. Marianne was great at this.

As we moved into the world of high technology, I had to learn new procedures to complete intakes and assessments online. I have no problem with learning new things, and no objection to using a computer, but I am still a bit of a paper person. Therefore, I start on paper cheat sheets and later enter the information onto the computer.

By this time, I was almost fifty years old and started looking at my life again. Was this job my final destiny? It had worked out well for the last seven years while my older child was starting out on his own and the younger two had so much going on in middle school and high school. My parents needed me more as my dad grew weaker with cancer and eventually died.

I missed being a real nurse. I love being busy, but I also knew I could not manage the vigorous physical work and mental stress of the hospital environment, or the need to work weekends and holidays. The work in home care could also be incredibly stressful and time-consuming.

CHAPTER 22 SUPERVISORY CHANGES

I thought about going to a clinic or doctor's office. I applied at two local doctors' offices and got calls back merely telling me I was overqualified.

I stayed connected with Brandy, my colleague from St. Christopher's ICU. She had been working for a law firm as a nurse paralegal for the past twelve years and was happy there. Until this point in my life, I really hadn't thought about working for lawyers, as medical staff and attorneys usually did not blend well.

Brandy and I had a long chat about her role. The place she worked was a defense firm, representing medical professionals. She said, "We are going to be seeking another nurse paralegal."

I thought this might be my new and final endeavor—and the firm's focus on health care workers would allow me to continue supporting my peers.

After updating my resume, I sent it to the firm's office manager. A few days later, I received a call asking me to come in for an interview early the following Monday morning.

That day I dressed in my blue suit and arrived at the very professional and somewhat formal office. A tall, slender young woman called me into a conference room, and as I walked toward the door, I felt butterflies such as I had not experienced at any other job interview.

Still, I got the job. My decision to move into the legal field was personal and might not suit every nurse. As I see it, I left the role of providing direct caregiving to one of supporting other caregivers. However, and wherever we serve, nurses provide the support people need to minimize distress and maximize wellness.

AUBREY LABALIA is a registered nurse who received her degree and license in the late 1970's and worked in various nursing roles as permitted by her license. Her employment included working in the medical surgical unit, intensive care unit, cardiac care unit, and the burn treatment unit in the hospital. Intermittently, she worked as a community health nurse and gravitated to the position an assessor nurse for an insurance program and finally entered the field as a legal nurse consultant.